Prologue

The moonlight filtered through the sheer curtains of the bedroom, casting a soft, silver glow over the room. Mia lay in bed, her hand resting gently on her stomach, a smile playing on her lips as she gazed up at the ceiling. The room was quiet, save for the occasional rustle of the sheets and the rhythmic ticking of the old clock on the nightstand.

Outside, the world seemed to hold its breath, wrapped in the tranquil stillness of the night. The city lights flickered in the distance, a reminder of the bustling life that continued beyond the calm of their home. Inside, the air was filled with a different kind of excitement, a quiet anticipation that had settled into the very fabric of their lives.

Mia's thoughts drifted back to the moment she had first held the tiny, fragile positive pregnancy test in her trembling hands. The news had come as a surprise, an unexpected twist in the journey she and Ethan had been on. For a moment, she had felt a mix of disbelief and wonder, her mind racing with a thousand questions and emotions.

But as the initial shock wore off, a deep sense of joy began to blossom within her. The realization that they were going to become parents filled her with a profound sense of hope and possibility. It was a joy that was both exhilarating and humbling, a gift that had arrived in the most unexpected of ways.

Ethan's excitement had been palpable when she had shared the news with him. His eyes had sparkled with a mix of disbelief and joy, and his embrace had been filled with a warmth that reassured her they were in this together. They had talked late into the night, dreaming of the future and envisioning the life they would build for their growing family.

In the quiet of the night, Mia felt a gentle fluttering, a reassuring reminder of the little life growing inside her. She closed her eyes, allowing herself to savor the moment. It was a feeling of connection and love that transcended words, a promise of the journey that lay ahead.

The road ahead was uncertain, filled with both challenges and joys. There would be moments of doubt and difficulty, but there would also be countless moments of wonder and love. Mia and Ethan were ready to embrace it all, knowing that their lives would be forever transformed by this unexpected joy.

As the moonlight bathed the room in its soft glow, Mia felt a deep sense of peace. The journey of parenthood was about to begin, and she was ready to face it with open hearts and unwavering commitment. She turned to Ethan, who was asleep beside her, and whispered softly, "We're going to be parents."

In the stillness of the night, Mia and Ethan's hearts beat in unison with the promise of new beginnings. The future was a blank canvas, waiting to be filled with the colors of their love, dreams, and hopes. With a heart full of joy and a spirit ready for the journey, Mia closed her eyes and drifted into a peaceful sleep, dreaming of the beautiful life that awaited them.

The prologue set the stage for the unfolding story, a tale of love, anticipation, and the unexpected blessings that life can bring. It was the beginning of a journey that would be filled with challenges, triumphs, and the simple, profound joy of watching their family grow.

Chapter 1: The News

Mia stared at the computer screen, her fingers hovering above the keyboard, the faint hum of the office filling the room. The cursor blinked, impatiently awaiting her next command. She had been working on this project for weeks, pouring over data, analyzing trends, and crafting the perfect presentation for the upcoming meeting with the board. This was her moment—the culmination of years of hard work and late nights.

But today, her mind was somewhere else, a distant place she couldn't quite reach. She rubbed her temples, trying to focus, but the nagging feeling in the pit of her stomach wouldn't go away. It wasn't just the nerves, it was something else, something she couldn't shake off.

The faint beep of her phone snapped her back to reality. She glanced at the screen—a reminder of the doctor's appointment she had almost forgotten about. It was just a routine check-up, nothing to worry about. She had been feeling off for a few weeks, but attributed it to stress and exhaustion. After all, she had been pushing herself to the limit with work, barely taking a moment to breathe.

Mia quickly saved her work, shut down the computer, and grabbed her coat. As she left the office, she caught a glimpse of herself in the mirror by the door—her usual sharp, confident appearance was slightly marred by the dark circles under her eyes and the hint of fatigue in her posture.

The drive to the doctor's office was a blur of honking horns and city lights. Mia's mind wandered as she tried to remember the last time she had felt truly relaxed. It had been months, maybe even years. Her life had become a series of deadlines and meetings, with little time for anything else. She had always prided herself on being independent and focused, but lately, she had started to wonder if she was missing out on something.

The waiting room was quiet, the soft murmur of conversations and the rustle of magazines filling the space. Mia checked in at the front desk and took a seat, her mind still racing. She pulled out her phone, scrolling through emails, trying to distract herself. But her thoughts kept drifting back to that nagging feeling, that sense that something was off.

"Ms. Anderson?" The nurse's voice pulled her out of her reverie. Mia looked up, nodded, and followed her down the hallway to the examination room.

The nurse took her vitals, made some small talk, and then left her alone to wait for the doctor. Mia tapped her fingers on the table, her anxiety growing. She hated waiting—she was a woman of action, always on the move, always in control. But here, in this sterile room, she felt vulnerable, exposed.

The door creaked open, and Dr. Patel walked in, her warm smile easing some of Mia's tension. She had been seeing Dr. Patel for years, trusting her with her health and well-being.

"Mia, how are you doing?" Dr. Patel asked, taking a seat across from her.

"I'm fine, just tired. Work's been crazy," Mia replied, brushing off the question with a smile.

Dr. Patel nodded, flipping through her chart. "You mentioned feeling off lately—can you tell me more about that?"

Mia hesitated, trying to find the right words. "I've just been really tired, more than usual. I thought it was just work stress, but it's been getting worse. And I've been feeling a bit nauseous in the mornings, but nothing too serious."

Dr. Patel looked at her thoughtfully, her pen tapping against the clipboard. "Have you been under a lot of stress lately? Any changes in your routine?"

Mia shrugged. "I guess so. Work's been intense, and I haven't been sleeping well. But that's nothing new."

Dr. Patel nodded again, then paused, her gaze softening. "Mia, I think it's a good idea to run a few tests, just to rule out anything serious. How's your cycle been?"

Mia blinked, caught off guard by the question. "My cycle? It's… I don't know, regular, I guess. I haven't really been paying attention."

Dr. Patel's expression grew more concerned. "When was your last period?"

Mia thought back, trying to remember, but the days and weeks had blurred together. "I think it was… about six weeks ago? Maybe longer."

Dr. Patel gave her a reassuring smile. "It's probably nothing, but let's just do a quick test to be sure."

Mia nodded, her heart starting to pound in her chest. She watched as Dr. Patel prepared the test, her movements calm and methodical. Mia tried to steady her breathing, telling herself it was just a precaution, nothing to worry about.

The minutes ticked by, each one feeling like an eternity. Mia's mind raced with a thousand thoughts, each one more frantic than the last. What if she was pregnant? What would that mean for her life, her career? She wasn't ready for this—she had plans, goals, things she wanted to accomplish before even thinking about starting a family.

Finally, Dr. Patel turned back to her, holding the test in her hand. Her expression was unreadable, and Mia felt her heart drop.

"Mia," Dr. Patel began, her voice gentle, "the test is positive."

The words hung in the air, heavy and unreal. Mia stared at her, not fully comprehending. "Positive? You mean… I'm pregnant?"

Dr. Patel nodded, her eyes filled with sympathy. "Yes, Mia. You're pregnant."

Mia felt the world shift beneath her feet. Everything she thought she knew, everything she had planned, suddenly felt uncertain, as if the ground had been pulled out from under her. She opened her mouth to speak, but no words came out. Her mind was a jumble of thoughts and emotions, none of them making sense.

Dr. Patel reached out, placing a comforting hand on Mia's arm. "I know this is a lot to take in. It's okay to feel overwhelmed. We can talk about your options, and I'm here to support you in whatever you decide."

Mia nodded numbly, her mind still struggling to catch up. Pregnant. She was pregnant. The word echoed in her mind, over and over, as if saying it enough times would make it real.

"I need… I need to think," Mia finally managed to say, her voice barely above a whisper.

"Of course," Dr. Patel said, her tone kind and understanding. "Take all the time you need. And remember, you don't have to go through this alone. There are resources and people who can help you."

Mia nodded again, her thoughts swirling. She barely registered the rest of the appointment, the words of advice and support from Dr. Patel. All she could think about was the tiny life growing inside her, a life she hadn't planned for, a life that changed everything.

The drive home was a blur. Mia couldn't focus on the road, her mind too consumed with the news she had just received. Pregnant. She was pregnant. How had this happened? She had always been careful, always made sure to take her birth control on time. But somewhere, something had gone wrong, and now she was facing a reality she had never imagined.

When she finally reached her apartment, Mia sat in the car for a long time, staring at the building in front of her. It felt strange, alien, as if it belonged to someone else. The life she had built, the life she had worked so hard for, suddenly felt distant, like a dream she was waking up from.

Mia slowly made her way up to her apartment, her movements robotic, her mind still in shock. When she opened the door, the familiar surroundings brought a small sense of comfort, but it was fleeting. She dropped her keys on the table, kicked off her shoes, and collapsed onto the couch, burying her face in her hands.

Tears welled up in her eyes, but she forced them back, trying to stay strong. She had always prided herself on her ability to handle anything life threw at her, but this… this was different. This was something she had never prepared for, something she had never even considered.

Mia's phone buzzed in her pocket, and she pulled it out, seeing a text from Lena, her best friend. *"How'd the doctor's appointment go? Everything okay?"*

Mia stared at the screen, her fingers trembling as she tried to type a response. But what could she say? How could she explain what she was feeling when she didn't even understand it herself?

Finally, she typed out a simple reply: *"I'm fine. Just tired."* It was a lie, but it was all she could manage. She couldn't bring herself to share the news, not yet. Not when she was still trying to process it herself.

As the evening wore on, Mia tried to distract herself with work, but the words on the screen blurred together, meaningless and distant. She couldn't focus, couldn't think about anything other than the tiny life growing inside her. She imagined what it would be like to have a child, to be responsible for another human being. The thought terrified her, but there was also a small flicker of something else, something she couldn't quite name.

The hours passed slowly, each one dragging on as Mia tried to come to terms with the reality of her situation. She knew she had to make a decision, but the weight of it felt overwhelming, crushing her under its enormity. She had always been so sure of her path, so certain of where she was going, but now… now everything was different.

As the night deepened, Mia finally allowed herself to cry. The tears came slowly at first, then faster, until she was sobbing uncontrollably, her body shaking with the force of it. She cried for the life she had planned, the life that was now slipping through her fingers. She cried for the fear and uncertainty that gripped her, for the sense of loss that she couldn't quite name.

When the tears finally subsided, Mia was left feeling drained, exhausted. But there was also a small sense of release, as if the tears had washed away some of the fear and confusion. She knew she still had a long way to go, still had decisions to make and challenges to face, but for the first time since hearing the news, she felt a tiny glimmer of hope.

Mia curled up on the couch, pulling a blanket over herself, and closed her eyes. She didn't know what the future held, didn't know what she would do or how she would manage. But she knew one thing for certain: she wasn't going to run from this. She would face it, whatever it was, and she would find a way to make it work.

As she drifted off to sleep, Mia's hand rested on her stomach, a subconscious gesture of protection and connection. For the first time since hearing the news, she allowed herself to think of the tiny life growing inside her, and what it might mean for her future.

The night was quiet, the only sound the soft hum of the city outside. And in that stillness, Mia began to imagine a new life, one that was unexpected, but perhaps, in some way, exactly what she needed.

Chapter 2: The Decision

Mia awoke the next morning feeling as though she had been run over by a truck. The night before had been a blur of emotion and confusion, and the heaviness of it all still weighed on her. She blinked her eyes open, the light filtering through the curtains casting a soft glow on her apartment, a place that had always been her sanctuary. But today, it felt different—less like a refuge and more like a reminder of the uncertainty she was facing.

She lay there for a long time, staring at the ceiling, her mind spinning with thoughts she couldn't quite catch. Her hand instinctively went to her stomach, resting there as if to confirm that it hadn't all been a bad dream. But it was real. She was pregnant. The word still felt foreign to her, like something that belonged to someone else's life, not hers.

The questions started to flood in again, just as they had the night before. What was she going to do? How could she possibly raise a child when her life was already so full, so complicated? Her career was everything to her, the one constant in a world that often felt chaotic and unpredictable. She had worked so hard to get where she was, to build a life she was proud of. And now, everything was in jeopardy.

Mia sat up slowly, pushing the blanket off her and swinging her legs over the side of the couch. She felt the coolness of the floor against her feet, grounding her in the present moment. The tears had dried, leaving behind a dull ache in her chest that she didn't know how to soothe. She wanted to cry again, but the tears wouldn't come. Instead, there was only a numbness, a feeling of being stuck in a place she couldn't escape.

She knew she had to make a decision. The thought terrified her, but there was no escaping it. She couldn't ignore this, couldn't pretend it wasn't happening. The life growing inside her was a reality she had to face, and the choices she made now would shape her future in ways she couldn't even begin to imagine.

But how could she decide? The options felt overwhelming, each one carrying its own set of challenges and consequences. She thought about all the things she wanted to do with her life—the places she wanted to go, the career milestones she wanted to achieve, the freedom she had always cherished. Would having a child mean giving all of that up? Would she be able to find a balance, or would she lose herself in the process?

Mia got up and walked to the kitchen, her movements slow and deliberate. She wasn't hungry, but she needed something to do, something to distract her from the thoughts swirling in her head. She made herself a cup of tea, the familiar routine offering a small measure of comfort. As she waited for the water to boil, she stared out the window, watching the city come to life outside.

The world was moving on, as it always did, indifferent to the turmoil inside her. People were going to work, living their lives, making decisions—big and small—that would shape their futures. And here she was, stuck in a moment she didn't know how to navigate.

The shrill whistle of the kettle broke her reverie, and she poured the hot water over the tea bag, watching as the liquid turned a deep amber. She took the cup to the table, sitting down and wrapping her hands around the warmth, letting it seep into her bones.

She knew she couldn't do this alone. She needed to talk to someone, to get some perspective, but the idea of sharing this news felt daunting. Who could she turn to? Lena, of course. Her best friend had always been there for her, through every up and down, every crisis and celebration. But would she understand? Would she be able to offer the support Mia needed, or would she see this as just another problem to solve?

Mia picked up her phone, hesitating for a moment before dialing Lena's number. Her heart pounded in her chest as she listened to the ringing on the other end.

Finally, Lena answered, her voice bright and cheerful as always. "Hey, Mia! What's up?"

Mia took a deep breath, trying to steady her nerves. "Hey, Lena. Do you have a minute? I... I really need to talk to you."

"Of course," Lena said, her tone immediately shifting to one of concern. "What's going on? Are you okay?"

Mia hesitated, the words catching in her throat. She had rehearsed this conversation in her head a dozen times, but now that it was actually happening, she didn't know where to start. "I... I went to the doctor yesterday," she began, her voice trembling slightly. "And I found out... I'm pregnant."

There was a long pause on the other end of the line, and for a moment, Mia wondered if Lena had hung up. But then she heard a soft intake of breath, followed by Lena's voice, now gentle and soothing. "Oh, Mia... I had no idea. How are you feeling?"

"I don't know," Mia admitted, her voice barely above a whisper. "I'm scared, Lena. I don't know what to do. This wasn't part of the plan."

Lena was silent for a moment, and when she spoke again, her voice was filled with empathy. "I can only imagine how overwhelming this must be for you. But you don't have to figure it all out right now. You don't have to make any decisions today. Just take it one step at a time."

Mia closed her eyes, letting Lena's words wash over her. She had been so caught up in the enormity of the situation that she had forgotten she didn't have to have all the answers immediately. Maybe it was okay to take a breath, to give herself the space to process what was happening.

"I just... I don't know if I'm ready for this," Mia said, her voice cracking with emotion. "My life is so busy, so full. I've worked so hard to get where I am. What if I can't do it all? What if I fail?"

Lena's voice was steady, reassuring. "Mia, you're one of the strongest, most capable people I know. If anyone can figure this out, it's you. But you don't have to do it alone. You have people who love you, who will support you no matter what you decide. And that includes me."

Mia felt a lump rise in her throat, the tears she had been holding back threatening to spill over. "Thank you, Lena. I don't know what I'd do without you."

"You'll never have to find out," Lena said softly. "Whatever you decide, I'm here for you, every step of the way."

They talked for a while longer, Lena offering words of comfort and understanding, helping Mia to see that she didn't have to have it all figured out right away. By the time they hung up, Mia felt a little more grounded, a little less overwhelmed. She still didn't know what she was going to do, but at least she knew she didn't have to face it alone.

After the call, Mia felt the need to get out of the apartment, to clear her head and try to find some clarity. She quickly dressed and grabbed her coat, deciding to take a walk through the nearby park. The fresh air might help her think, and the familiar paths could offer some solace.

The park was a place Mia often visited when she needed to escape the pressures of life. It was her sanctuary, a place where she could breathe and let her mind wander. As she walked, the cool breeze brushed against her face, and the sound of leaves crunching underfoot brought a small sense of peace. The park was quiet this morning, with only a few joggers and dog walkers passing by, each absorbed in their own world.

Mia found herself drawn to a small bench near the edge of the park, where the trees opened up to reveal a view of the city skyline. She sat down, her thoughts still swirling but beginning to settle. She watched the city in the distance, its buildings standing tall and unyielding, a testament to the strength and determination she had always admired.

But even as she looked at the skyline, Mia couldn't help but think about the tiny life growing inside her. It was so small, so fragile, yet it had the power to change everything. She wondered what it would be like to be a mother, to hold her child in her arms and feel the bond that so many others had described. It was a role she had never envisioned for herself, yet now, she couldn't stop thinking about it.

Mia's thoughts turned to her own childhood, to the memories of her mother and father, who had always been there for her, supporting her dreams and encouraging her to be whoever she wanted to be. They had given her the foundation to build the life she had, and she wondered if she could do the same for her own child. Could she offer that same unwavering support and love, even if it meant putting her own dreams on hold?

The thought scared her, but it also stirred something deep within her, something she hadn't expected. It wasn't just fear or uncertainty—it was a longing, a desire to connect with this new life in a way that she had never imagined. Maybe, just maybe, this was an opportunity to find a new kind of fulfillment, one that went beyond career success or personal achievements.

As the sun began to rise higher in the sky, Mia felt a sense of clarity beginning to emerge. She didn't have all the answers, but she knew she had to trust herself, to believe that she could handle whatever came her way. She had always been strong, always found a way to succeed, and this would be no different. Yes, it would be challenging, and yes, it would change everything, but maybe that wasn't such a bad thing.

Mia knew she needed to talk to someone else, someone who could offer more perspective. She thought about her parents, who had always been a source of wisdom and guidance. They had supported her through every decision she had ever made, even when they didn't fully understand her choices. They would listen, and they would offer their advice, but they would also respect whatever decision she made.

She pulled out her phone and dialed her mother's number, her heart pounding as she waited for her to pick up. When her mother's familiar voice answered, Mia felt a rush of emotion, the tears she had been holding back threatening to spill over.

"Hi, Mom," she said, her voice trembling slightly.

"Mia, sweetheart, it's so good to hear from you! How are you doing?" her mother asked, her voice warm and full of love.

"I'm... I'm okay," Mia said, struggling to find the right words. "But I need to talk to you about something. Something important."

There was a pause on the other end, and Mia could almost hear the concern in her mother's voice when she spoke again. "Of course, honey. What's going on?"

Mia took a deep breath, the words finally tumbling out. "I'm pregnant, Mom. I found out yesterday, and... I don't know what to do."

Her mother was silent for a moment, and when she spoke again, her voice was filled with compassion. "Oh, Mia... I'm sure this is a lot to take in. But whatever you decide, I want you to know that your father and I are here for you. We love you, and we'll support you no matter what."

Mia felt a wave of relief wash over her, the weight of the decision feeling just a little bit lighter. "Thank you, Mom. I'm so scared, and I don't know if I'm ready for this. I've worked so hard for my career, and I'm worried that I'll have to give it all up."

Her mother's voice was soothing, filled with the wisdom that only years of experience could bring. "Mia, being a mother is one of the most challenging and rewarding things you'll ever do, but it doesn't mean you have to give up your dreams. You're strong, capable, and determined. You can find a way to balance it all. It won't be easy, but nothing worth doing ever is."

Mia listened to her mother's words, letting them sink in. Her mother had always been her rock, the one she turned to in times of doubt and fear. And now, more than ever, she needed that support. "I don't want to make a decision out of fear," Mia said, her voice steadying. "But I also don't want to make a decision I'll regret."

Her mother's voice was filled with understanding. "It's okay to be afraid, Mia. It's okay to not have all the answers right now. But whatever you choose, make sure it's a decision that feels right in your heart. You have a good head on your shoulders, and I trust that you'll make the right choice for you."

Mia nodded, even though her mother couldn't see her. "Thank you, Mom. I just needed to hear that."

"Anytime, sweetheart," her mother replied, her voice filled with love. "And remember, you don't have to go through this alone. Your father and I are here, Lena is there, and you have so many people who care about you. Lean on them when you need to.”

Mia felt a sense of calm wash over her, a feeling of being held by the people who loved her most. “I will, Mom. Thank you.”

They talked for a little while longer, her mother offering more words of wisdom and support, helping Mia to see that she didn’t have to make a decision out of fear or pressure. She could take her time, weigh her options, and trust that whatever she chose, it would be the right choice for her.

After hanging up, Mia sat on the bench for a long time, letting the conversation with her mother replay in her mind. Her mother’s words had given her a sense of peace, a feeling that she could handle whatever came her way. She didn’t have to make a decision right now, and she didn’t have to do it alone. She had the support of the people who loved her, and she had her own inner strength to guide her.

Mia knew that the path ahead wouldn’t be easy, but she also knew that she was capable of facing it. She had faced challenges before, and she had always come out stronger on the other side. This would be no different. She would take it one step at a time, trusting herself and the people around her to help her find her way.

As she got up from the bench and began to walk back through the park, Mia felt a sense of resolve forming within her. She didn't have all the answers yet, but she knew she would find them. She would make the right decision for herself, and whatever that decision was, she would embrace it fully.

The city skyline loomed in the distance, a reminder of the life she had built and the dreams she had worked so hard to achieve. But now, there was something new, something unexpected, blossoming in her life. And for the first time since hearing the news, Mia felt a sense of possibility, a feeling that maybe this wasn't the end of her dreams, but the beginning of something even greater.

She walked back to her apartment with a new sense of purpose, knowing that whatever decision she made, it would be hers and hers alone. She would find a way to make it work, to balance her career, her dreams, and the new life growing inside her. And she would do it with the strength and determination that had always defined her.

As she opened the door to her apartment, Mia took a deep breath, feeling the weight of the decision still ahead of her, but also feeling a sense of peace she hadn't had before. She would take her time, trust herself, and know that whatever she chose, it would be the right decision for her and her future.

Chapter 3: Telling the Father

The days following Mia's conversation with her mother were a mix of reflection and determination. She spent time thinking about her life, her future, and the decisions that lay ahead. She knew she couldn't delay forever, and there was one person she hadn't yet spoken to—Ethan, the father of her unborn child. The thought of telling him filled her with anxiety, but it was a conversation she knew she couldn't avoid.

Mia had met Ethan a year earlier at a mutual friend's party. He was charming, with a quick wit and an easy smile that drew people to him. Their connection had been instant, a spark that turned into something more over time. They had kept things casual, neither of them ready for anything serious, but there had always been a deep respect and understanding between them. Now, everything had changed.

The reality of the situation weighed heavily on her as she tried to figure out how to approach the conversation. How would Ethan react? Would he be shocked, angry, or supportive? Would he want to be involved, or would he see this as a burden?

These questions plagued her, and the uncertainty gnawed at her insides.

She spent the morning pacing her apartment, trying to muster the courage to make the call. Her hand hovered over her phone more than once, but she couldn't bring herself to dial his number. The fear of the unknown was paralyzing. What if this changed everything between them? What if he didn't want anything to do with her or the baby? The thought was unbearable, but Mia knew she couldn't let fear dictate her actions.

Finally, as the afternoon sun cast long shadows across her living room, Mia forced herself to pick up the phone. She scrolled through her contacts until she found Ethan's name, her heart pounding as she pressed the call button. The phone rang once, twice, three times, and Mia's nerves grew with each passing second.

When Ethan finally answered, his voice was warm and familiar, instantly bringing back memories of their time together. "Hey, Mia! It's been a while. How've you been?"

Mia swallowed hard, trying to keep her voice steady. "Hi, Ethan. I'm… I'm okay. How about you?"

"I'm good, just busy with work, you know how it is. It's really great to hear from you. What's up?" His tone was casual, as if nothing had changed, as if this was just another friendly call between two people who had shared something special.

Mia felt a lump in her throat, the weight of what she was about to say pressing down on her. "Ethan, there's something I need to talk to you about. It's… it's important."

There was a pause on the other end, and when Ethan spoke again, his voice was more serious. "Okay, you're starting to worry me. What's going on?"

Mia took a deep breath, forcing herself to get the words out. "Ethan, I found out a few days ago that… I'm pregnant."

The silence that followed was deafening. Mia could almost hear the gears turning in Ethan's mind as he processed what she had just said. She held her breath, waiting for his response, her heart pounding in her chest.

Finally, Ethan spoke, his voice tinged with shock. "You're… you're pregnant? Are you sure?"

"Yes, I'm sure," Mia replied, her voice barely above a whisper. "I've been to the doctor. It's real, Ethan. I'm pregnant."

Another long pause. Mia could feel the tension between them, the uncertainty and fear that had suddenly become all too real. She wanted to say something, anything, to break the silence, but she didn't know what to say. This was uncharted territory, a situation neither of them had ever imagined.

When Ethan finally spoke again, his voice was softer, more measured. "Wow… I don't even know what to say. This is… unexpected, to say the least."

Mia nodded, even though he couldn't see her. "I know. It's a lot to take in. I've been trying to process it myself, but I knew I had to tell you. You deserve to know."

"Yeah, of course," Ethan said, his voice thoughtful. "I just… I wasn't expecting this. We were always careful, you know? But I guess nothing's ever foolproof."

Mia felt a pang of guilt at his words. They had been careful, but clearly, something had gone wrong. It wasn't anyone's fault, but that didn't make it any easier to accept. "I know, Ethan. This isn't what either of us planned, but it's happening. And we need to figure out what to do next."

Ethan was silent for a moment, as if weighing his options. When he spoke again, his voice was filled with uncertainty. "What are you thinking, Mia? Have you made any decisions yet?"

Mia hesitated, the enormity of the situation crashing down on her once again. "I've been thinking about it a lot, but I haven't made any final decisions. I wanted to talk to you first, to see how you feel about all of this."

"How I feel?" Ethan echoed, as if the question had caught him off guard. "I… I don't know, Mia. This is huge. I never imagined I'd be having this conversation, especially not now. But… I guess we need to figure it out together."

His words brought a small measure of relief to Mia. At least he wasn't shutting down or running away. He was willing to have the conversation, to be a part of this, whatever "this" turned out to be. "I appreciate that, Ethan. I know this isn't easy, but I want us to be on the same page, whatever we decide."

"Yeah, of course," Ethan agreed. "We'll figure it out, Mia. We have to. But I need some time to process this, to wrap my head around it. This is a lot to take in."

"I understand," Mia said, her voice gentle. "I needed time too. This wasn't something I could just… accept right away. But I'm here, Ethan. We can talk whenever you're ready."

"Thanks, Mia," Ethan said, his voice sincere. "I'm really glad you told me. I wouldn't want you to go through this alone."

Mia felt a surge of emotion at his words. She had been so afraid of telling him, so worried about how he would react, but his response had been more understanding than she had dared to hope. "I'm glad I told you too. We're in this together, Ethan, no matter what happens."

They talked a little longer, the conversation gradually shifting away from the initial shock and toward a more practical discussion of what came next. Ethan asked questions—about the pregnancy, about how Mia was feeling, about the future—and Mia answered as best she could, though many of the answers were still unclear.

By the time they hung up, Mia felt a mixture of emotions—relief, anxiety, and a strange sense of calm. The conversation had gone better than she had feared, but it was clear that there were still many unknowns, many challenges ahead. Still, she was grateful that Ethan was willing to be a part of the journey, whatever it might bring.

The next few days passed in a blur of introspection and contemplation. Mia and Ethan spoke several times, each conversation helping to clarify their thoughts and feelings. They discussed the practicalities—finances, living arrangements, the impact on their careers—but also the emotional aspects, the fears and hopes that came with the territory.

Mia found herself thinking a lot about what kind of father Ethan would be. He was kind, intelligent, and responsible, but fatherhood was a completely different kind of responsibility. Would he rise to the occasion, or would the pressure become too much? She knew she couldn't predict the future, but she couldn't help wondering how this would all play out.

Ethan, for his part, was grappling with his own set of emotions. He had never seen himself as the fatherly type, at least not at this point in his life. He enjoyed his freedom, his career, and the casual nature of his relationship with Mia. But now, everything was changing, and he had to figure out what that meant for him. Could he step up to the role of father, or would he falter under the weight of the responsibility?

As the days turned into a week, Ethan called Mia and suggested they meet in person. "We need to talk face-to-face," he said. "There's only so much we can figure out over the phone."

Mia agreed, knowing that this was a conversation that couldn't be had over a phone line. They arranged to meet at a quiet café they both liked, a place where they could talk without interruptions. Mia felt a knot of anxiety in her stomach as she made her way to the café, the gravity of the situation pressing down on her. This meeting felt pivotal, like a turning point in their lives.

When she arrived at the café, she found Ethan already seated at a table near the back, a coffee cup in front of him. He looked up as she approached, giving her a small, reassuring smile that did little to calm her nerves. She sat down across from him, her heart pounding in her chest.

"Hey," Ethan said, his voice gentle. "Thanks for meeting me."

"Of course," Mia replied, trying to keep her voice steady. "We need to talk."

"Yeah, we do," Ethan agreed, his expression serious. He took a deep breath, as if gathering his thoughts. "Mia, I've been doing a lot of thinking since we talked. This whole situation… it's overwhelming. But I want you to know that I'm here. I'm not going to disappear or leave you to deal with this on your own."

Mia felt a wave of relief at his words, but she also knew that this was just the beginning. There was so much more they needed to discuss, so many decisions that still needed to be made. "I'm really glad to hear that, Ethan. But we still need to figure out what this means for us, for the baby, for our lives."

Ethan nodded, his expression thoughtful. "I know. I've been thinking a lot about that too. And I've come to the conclusion that… I want to be involved. I want to be a part of this baby's life, if that's what you want too."

Mia felt a surge of emotion at his words. This was what she had hoped for, what she had feared might not happen. But hearing him say it out loud made it real, and that brought its own set of challenges. "I do want that, Ethan. I want us to figure this out together. But it's not going to be easy. We both have our lives, our careers, and this is going to change everything."

"I know," Ethan said, his voice steady. "But I'm willing to make those changes, to figure out how to make this work. I don't want to walk away from this, Mia. I want to be there for you, and for our child."

Mia felt tears prick at the corners of her eyes. She had been so afraid of this conversation, so worried that Ethan wouldn't want to be involved, that he would see this as a burden rather than a responsibility. But here he was, offering his support, his commitment, and it filled her with a sense of hope.

"Thank you, Ethan," she said, her voice choked with emotion. "That means so much to me. I've been so scared, so unsure of what to do, but knowing that you're here… it makes a difference."

Ethan reached across the table and took her hand, his touch warm and reassuring. "We'll figure this out, Mia. We don't have all the answers yet, but we'll find them together. We're in this together, okay?"

Mia nodded, squeezing his hand. "Okay."

They spent the next few hours talking, sharing their fears, hopes, and uncertainties. They discussed the practicalities—how they would balance their careers with raising a child, where they would live, how they would handle finances. But they also talked about the emotional aspects—the impact this would have on their relationship, the kind of parents they wanted to be, and the future they envisioned for their child.

By the time they left the café, Mia felt a sense of resolve she hadn't felt before. This wasn't going to be easy, but they were committed to making it work. They had taken the first steps toward a new chapter in their lives, and while the road ahead was uncertain, they knew they wouldn't be walking it alone.

As she walked back to her apartment, Mia couldn't help but feel a sense of relief. The conversation had gone better than she could have hoped, and while there were still many challenges ahead, she felt a renewed sense of hope and determination.

They would figure this out, one step at a time, and they would do it together.

Ethan's commitment to being involved, to facing this challenge with her, had given her the strength she needed to move forward. She knew there would be difficult days ahead, but she also knew that they could handle it, as long as they faced it together.

As Mia opened the door to her apartment, she took a deep breath, feeling a sense of peace settle over her. This was the beginning of something new, something unexpected, but also something filled with possibility. She didn't have all the answers yet, but she was ready to face whatever came next, with Ethan by her side.

Chapter 4: Facing Family

After the conversation with Ethan, Mia felt like a weight had been lifted from her shoulders. The uncertainty that had plagued her since discovering the pregnancy was still there, but it was tempered by the knowledge that she wasn't alone in this. Ethan's commitment to being involved and supportive gave her a renewed sense of strength, but she knew that the journey ahead was still fraught with challenges. One of the biggest hurdles would be facing their families.

Mia's relationship with her parents was close, built on a foundation of mutual respect and understanding. They had always supported her, even when her choices didn't align with their expectations. However, this was different. Mia was acutely aware of the hopes and dreams her parents had for her—hopes that didn't necessarily include an unplanned pregnancy. The thought of disappointing them gnawed at her, even though she knew they would ultimately stand by her.

The decision to tell her parents weighed heavily on Mia's mind. She had spoken to her mother briefly after learning the news, but that conversation had been more about seeking comfort than confronting the reality of the situation. Now, with Ethan on board, it was time to have a more serious discussion. She dreaded the idea of seeing the look of shock, or perhaps even disappointment, on her parents' faces. But it had to be done.

Mia decided to tell her parents over dinner, hoping that the familiar setting of their home might make the conversation easier. As she drove to their house, her mind raced with possible scenarios, rehearsing what she might say and how they might react. The closer she got, the more her anxiety grew, until she was practically trembling by the time she pulled into their driveway.

Her parents greeted her warmly at the door, her mother's arms wrapping around her in a comforting hug. "Mia, sweetheart, it's so good to see you! It feels like ages since we've had you over for dinner."

Mia smiled, though it felt strained. "I know, Mom. I've been so busy with work and everything."

Her father joined them in the hallway, giving her a quick kiss on the forehead. "Busy is good, but it's even better to have you here with us tonight."

Mia followed her parents into the kitchen, where the familiar smells of her mother's cooking filled the air. She tried to focus on the present moment, the warmth of her parents' home, the comfort of being with them. But the knowledge of what she needed to say hung over her like a cloud, making it hard to fully relax.

As they sat down to dinner, her mother began to chatter about the latest neighborhood gossip, filling the silence with stories of the neighbors and their lives. Her father chimed in occasionally, adding his own commentary, but Mia remained mostly silent, her thoughts elsewhere. She picked at her food, barely tasting it, her mind consumed with how she would break the news.

Finally, as the conversation lulled, Mia realized that the moment had come. She couldn't put it off any longer. Clearing her throat, she looked up at her parents, her heart pounding in her chest.

"Mom, Dad… there's something I need to talk to you about," she began, her voice trembling slightly.

Her parents exchanged a glance, their expressions immediately shifting to concern. "What is it, sweetheart?" her mother asked, her tone gentle.

Mia took a deep breath, trying to steady herself. "I'm pregnant."

The words hung in the air, heavy and laden with meaning. Her parents stared at her in stunned silence, the shock evident on their faces. Her mother's hand flew to her mouth, her eyes wide, while her father's expression hardened with worry.

"Pregnant?" her father echoed, his voice laced with disbelief. "Mia, are you sure?"

"Yes, I'm sure," Mia replied, her voice barely above a whisper. "I've been to the doctor. I'm about eight weeks along."

Her mother lowered her hand from her mouth, her eyes filling with tears. "Oh, Mia… this is so unexpected. I don't know what to say."

Mia could feel the tension in the room, the weight of their emotions pressing down on her. She knew they weren't angry, but the shock and concern in their eyes was almost harder to bear. "I know this isn't what you expected," she said, her voice faltering. "It's not what I expected either. But it's happening, and I'm going to need your support."

Her father leaned back in his chair, his brow furrowed in thought. "Mia, we love you, and we'll always support you. But this is… a lot to take in. Have you thought about what this means for your career, your future?"

Mia nodded, feeling a lump in her throat. "Yes, I've thought about it a lot. And it's not going to be easy. But I've talked to Ethan, and he's willing to be involved, to help me figure this out. We're not sure what the future holds, but we're going to face it together."

Her mother reached across the table, taking Mia's hand in hers. "Mia, we're here for you, no matter what. We just want what's best for you. This is going to change everything, but you don't have to go through it alone."

Tears welled up in Mia's eyes at her mother's words, the relief and gratitude overwhelming her. "Thank you, Mom. I'm so scared, but knowing that you're here… it makes a difference."

Her father, who had been quiet up until now, finally spoke again, his voice softening. "We just want to make sure you're thinking this through, Mia. This is a big responsibility, and it's going to affect every part of your life. But if this is what you want, we'll support you every step of the way."

Mia nodded, her tears spilling over. "I know it's going to be hard, but I've made up my mind. I'm going to have this baby."

Her parents exchanged another glance, their expressions softening with acceptance. "Then we'll be here for you, whatever you need," her mother said, her voice filled with love. "You're our daughter, Mia, and we'll always be here for you."

The conversation continued, with her parents asking more questions—about Ethan, about the pregnancy, about her plans. Mia answered as best she could, though many of the answers were still unclear. But the tension in the room had eased, replaced by a sense of unity and support. Mia knew that her parents were still processing the news, but their love and commitment to her was unwavering.

As the evening wore on, Mia felt a sense of relief settle over her. The conversation had been difficult, but it had gone better than she had feared. Her parents were shocked, yes, but they were also supportive and loving, just as they had always been. And knowing that she had their backing gave her the strength she needed to face the challenges ahead.

But Mia knew that this was only half of the battle. There was still another family to face—Ethan's.

Unlike her own family, Mia's relationship with Ethan's parents was more distant. They had met a few times, mostly at social gatherings, but she had never formed a close bond with them. Ethan's parents were kind and polite, but there was always a sense of formality in their interactions, a subtle distance that made Mia feel like an outsider.

The thought of telling Ethan's parents about the pregnancy filled Mia with anxiety. She wasn't sure how they would react, especially given that she and Ethan weren't married or even in a serious relationship. Would they see her as a burden, a complication in their son's life? Would they support Ethan's decision to be involved, or would they pressure him to distance himself from the situation?

Mia discussed her concerns with Ethan, and he reassured her that his parents would ultimately come around. "They'll be shocked, sure," he admitted. "But they'll support us. They just need time to process it, like everyone else."

They decided to tell Ethan's parents together, hoping that a united front would help ease the shock. The night before the planned dinner with his parents, Mia could hardly sleep, her mind racing with all the possible outcomes. She couldn't shake the feeling of dread, the fear that this conversation might not go as smoothly as the one with her own parents.

The next day, Mia and Ethan drove to his parents' house, the car ride filled with nervous tension. Ethan tried to keep the mood light, making small talk and cracking jokes, but Mia could tell that he was just as anxious as she was. They were stepping into the unknown, and the uncertainty was overwhelming.

When they arrived at his parents' house, Mia's heart was pounding in her chest. Ethan's parents greeted them warmly at the door, his mother enveloping them in a hug. "It's so good to see you both! It's been too long," she said, her voice cheerful and welcoming.

Ethan's father, a reserved man with a quiet demeanor, nodded in agreement. "Yes, it's always nice to have you here."

Mia forced a smile, trying to match their warmth, but the anxiety gnawed at her insides. They made their way into the living room, where drinks and appetizers were waiting. Ethan's parents made small talk, asking about work and life in the city, but Mia found it hard to focus on the conversation. Her mind was elsewhere, consumed with what was to come.

After what felt like an eternity, Ethan finally cleared his throat, signaling that it was time to shift the conversation. "Mom, Dad, there's something Mia and I need to talk to you about," he began, his voice steady but serious.

His parents exchanged a glance, their expressions immediately shifting to concern. "What is it, Ethan?" his mother asked, her tone cautious.

Ethan took a deep breath, his hand squeezing Mia's for reassurance. "Mia is pregnant."

The room fell into stunned silence, the weight of the news settling over them like a thick fog. Ethan's parents stared at him in shock, their expressions a mix of surprise, confusion, and concern. Mia felt the tension in the room grow, the anxiety tightening in her chest.

"Pregnant?" Ethan's mother finally said, her voice barely above a whisper. "Are you sure?"

"Yes, we're sure," Ethan replied, his voice firm. "We've been to the doctor, and Mia's about eight weeks along."

Ethan's father leaned forward, his expression serious. "This is... unexpected. What are you planning to do?"

Mia could feel the weight of their scrutiny, the unspoken questions hanging in the air. She knew that this was a pivotal moment, one that would determine how their relationship with Ethan's parents would unfold. She took a deep breath, trying to steady her nerves.

"We've talked about it a lot," Mia began, her voice trembling slightly. "And we've decided that we're going to have this baby. We're not sure what the future holds, but we're committed to figuring it out together."

Ethan's mother's eyes filled with tears, her expression a mix of emotions. "Oh, Ethan... Mia... this is such a big decision. Are you sure you're ready for this? It's going to change everything."

Ethan nodded, his hand still tightly gripping Mia's. "We know it's going to be hard, but we're ready to face it. We need your support, though. This is going to be a challenge, and we can't do it alone."

Ethan's father remained silent, his brow furrowed in thought. Finally, he spoke, his voice measured.

"This is a big responsibility, Ethan. It's going to require a lot of sacrifices, and it's not something to be taken lightly."

"We understand that, Dad," Ethan replied, his tone respectful but resolute. "But we're committed to making it work. This wasn't planned, but it's happening, and we're going to do everything we can to make sure our child has a good life."

Ethan's mother reached out and placed a hand on Mia's arm, her touch gentle. "Mia, you must be feeling so overwhelmed. This is a lot to take in, and I'm sure you're scared. But we're here for you, just as we're here for Ethan. We'll support you both, whatever you need."

Tears welled up in Mia's eyes at her words, the relief washing over her like a wave. "Thank you," she whispered, her voice choked with emotion. "I was so afraid… but knowing that you're here means so much to me."

Ethan's parents exchanged a look, their expressions softening with acceptance. "We're still processing this," Ethan's father said, his voice gentle. "But we love you both, and we'll do whatever we can to help you through this. You're family, and we'll face this together."

The conversation continued, with Ethan's parents asking more questions—about their plans, their living arrangements, their thoughts on parenting. Mia and Ethan answered as best they could, though many of the details were still up in the air. But the tension in the room had eased, replaced by a sense of unity and support.

As the evening wore on, Mia felt a sense of relief and gratitude. The conversation had been difficult, but it had gone better than she had feared. Ethan's parents were shocked, yes, but they were also supportive and loving, just as she had hoped they would be. And knowing that they had the backing of both sets of parents gave Mia and Ethan the strength they needed to face the challenges ahead.

By the time they left Ethan's parents' house, Mia felt a sense of calm she hadn't experienced since discovering the pregnancy. The road ahead was still uncertain, but she knew that she and Ethan wouldn't be walking it alone. They had the support of their families, and that made all the difference.

As they drove home, Mia and Ethan talked about the evening, reflecting on how their parents had reacted and what it meant for their future. They knew there would be more difficult conversations ahead, more challenges to face, but they also knew that they had a solid foundation of love and support to build on.

Mia felt a renewed sense of hope as they pulled into her apartment complex. The conversations with their families had been a turning point, a moment of truth that had solidified their commitment to each other and to their unborn child. They were no longer just two individuals facing an unexpected situation—they were a team, with the love and support of their families behind them.

As Mia climbed into bed that night, she felt a sense of peace that had eluded her for weeks. The future was still uncertain, but for the first time, she felt ready to face it. She had Ethan by her side, and together, they would navigate the challenges ahead. With the love of their families and their own determination, they would find a way to make this unexpected journey one filled with joy and possibility.

And as she drifted off to sleep, Mia allowed herself to dream of the future—not with fear, but with hope. The path ahead was still unclear, but she knew that they would find their way, one step at a time, with the support of those who loved them most.

Chapter 5: Navigating Changes

The reality of impending parenthood settled in slowly for Mia and Ethan, like the dawning of a quiet morning, where the sky gradually shifts from night to day. Initially, the changes in Mia's body were subtle—a little extra fatigue, a hint of nausea, a growing sensitivity to smells. But as the weeks passed, those changes became more pronounced, forcing them to confront the profound transformation their lives were undergoing.

Mia was the first to feel the weight of these changes. The first trimester had been challenging—her energy levels dipped dramatically, and the morning sickness, which often struck at any time of the day, made it difficult for her to maintain her usual pace. Mia had always been someone who thrived on routine, on the predictability of her days, but now, her body dictated the rhythm of her life, and it was an unpredictable maestro.

She began to struggle with her job. As a project manager at a marketing firm, Mia was used to juggling multiple tasks, managing tight deadlines, and coordinating with various teams. But now, just getting through the workday was a challenge.

Meetings that once energized her now drained her, and by mid-afternoon, she often found herself fighting to stay awake at her desk. The exhaustion was bone-deep, and the nausea, while less frequent than in the early weeks, still lurked in the background, ready to pounce at the slightest provocation.

One afternoon, after a particularly grueling day, Mia found herself sitting in her car in the office parking lot, her hands gripping the steering wheel as she tried to muster the energy to drive home. She stared out the windshield, the world beyond the glass seeming distant and unreal. The thought of the drive home, the traffic, the noise, and the effort it would take to cook dinner and keep up the façade of normalcy was overwhelming.

Mia's phone buzzed in her bag, snapping her out of her daze. It was Ethan, texting to check in on her. His concern was a constant source of comfort, but today, it also brought a wave of guilt. She had been short with him lately, her patience worn thin by the physical and emotional toll of pregnancy. But Ethan, bless him, never complained. He simply stepped up, taking on more of the household chores, cooking dinner most nights, and making sure Mia had what she needed to feel comfortable.

But Mia could see the strain in his eyes, the way he sometimes stared off into the distance, lost in thought. He was trying so hard to be strong for her, to be the rock she could lean on, but she knew this was hard for him too. They were both navigating uncharted waters, and it was easy to lose sight of each other amidst the swirling currents of their own anxieties.

When Mia finally walked through the door that evening, she found Ethan in the kitchen, chopping vegetables for dinner. The sight of him, so domestic and focused, brought tears to her eyes. She hadn't realized how much she had come to rely on him, how much she had taken his support for granted.

"Hey," Ethan said, looking up from his task and smiling when he saw her. "How was your day?"

Mia dropped her bag by the door and walked over to him, wrapping her arms around his waist from behind and resting her head against his back. "Long," she murmured. "I'm so tired, Ethan. I don't know how much longer I can keep up with work."

Ethan put down the knife and turned to face her, concern etched into his features. "Mia, you've been pushing yourself too hard. You need to take care of yourself, and the baby. Maybe it's time to talk to your boss about reducing your hours, or even taking some time off."

Mia sighed, pulling away to lean against the counter. "I know you're right, but it's so hard. I've worked so hard to get where I am, and I don't want to let anyone down."

"You're not letting anyone down," Ethan said gently, reaching out to take her hand. "Your health, and the baby's health, are the most important things right now. Work will still be there when you're ready to go back."

Mia knew he was right, but that didn't make the decision any easier. The next day, she scheduled a meeting with her boss to discuss her options. It was a difficult conversation, one that left her feeling vulnerable and uncertain. But her boss was understanding, and together, they came up with a plan that allowed Mia to work from home part-time and reduce her hours. It was a relief, but it also marked the beginning of a new reality for Mia—one where she had to learn to let go, to accept that she couldn't do everything, at least not in the way she used to.

Ethan, meanwhile, was facing his own challenges at work. The company he worked for was in the midst of a major project, and the pressure was mounting. Ethan was used to handling stress, but this was different. The stakes felt higher now, with a baby on the way, and the added responsibility weighed heavily on him. He found himself working late into the night, trying to meet deadlines while also making sure he was there for Mia.

One night, after another long day at the office, Ethan came home to find Mia asleep on the couch, a book resting on her chest. She looked so peaceful, her features softened by sleep, and for a moment, Ethan just stood there, watching her. The sight of her like this, so vulnerable and yet so strong, filled him with a fierce protectiveness.

He knelt beside the couch, gently brushing a strand of hair from her face. Mia stirred, her eyes fluttering open. "Ethan," she murmured, blinking sleepily. "What time is it?"

"Late," Ethan replied, his voice soft. "I didn't mean to wake you."

Mia smiled, reaching out to take his hand. "You're home now. That's all that matters."

Ethan's heart ached at her words. He knew he hadn't been as present as he wanted to be, that his work was pulling him in directions he didn't want to go. But hearing Mia say that, seeing the love and trust in her eyes, made him realize how much she needed him, how much he needed to be there for her.

They stayed like that for a while, holding hands in the quiet of the living room, the world outside fading away. It was moments like this that reminded Ethan of what really mattered, that gave him the strength to keep going.

As the pregnancy progressed, Mia and Ethan began to make more concrete preparations for the baby's arrival. They started with the nursery, turning the spare room into a cozy, welcoming space. Mia took the lead on decorating, choosing soft colors and whimsical designs, while Ethan handled the more practical aspects, like assembling the crib and installing shelves.

The nursery became a symbol of their new life together, a tangible representation of the changes they were undergoing. Every time Mia walked into the room, she felt a mix of emotions—excitement, fear, love, and anticipation. It was overwhelming at times, but it also grounded her, reminding her that this journey, however challenging, was leading to something beautiful.

They also began to tackle the financial aspect of having a baby, a task that proved to be more daunting than either of them had anticipated. The costs associated with pregnancy, childbirth, and raising a child quickly added up, and they spent many evenings going over their budget, trying to figure out how to make it work.

Ethan took on extra work, picking up freelance projects in the evenings and on weekends. It was exhausting, but he knew they needed the extra money. Mia, too, found ways to contribute, selling some of her old clothes and belongings online and cutting back on non-essential expenses. It wasn't easy, but they were determined to provide the best for their baby.

Despite the financial strain, they found joy in the process of preparing for their baby. They spent weekends visiting thrift stores and garage sales, looking for gently used baby furniture and clothes. Mia's friends and family also pitched in, throwing a baby shower that left them well-stocked with essentials.

One Saturday, as they were putting the finishing touches on the nursery, Mia stood back and looked around the room, her hands resting on her belly. "It's really happening, isn't it?" she said, her voice tinged with awe.

Ethan came up behind her, wrapping his arms around her waist and resting his chin on her shoulder. "Yeah," he murmured. "It really is."

They stood there for a long time, taking it all in. The room was ready, and soon, so would they be. The changes they had navigated together—the physical, emotional, and practical challenges—had brought them closer than ever. They had learned to lean on each other, to communicate openly, and to find joy in the small moments.

But as prepared as they felt, they knew that the biggest changes were still to come. The arrival of their baby would turn their lives upside down in ways they couldn't fully anticipate. And yet, in that moment, standing in the nursery they had created together, they felt ready—ready to face whatever challenges lay ahead, ready to embrace the joy and chaos of parenthood, and ready to welcome their baby into the world.

The weeks passed in a blur of activity and anticipation. Mia's belly grew rounder, her movements slower, and her emotions more intense. Ethan was by her side through it all, holding her hand during doctor's appointments, rubbing her back when she was uncomfortable, and making late-night runs to satisfy her cravings.

As they entered the final weeks of pregnancy, the reality of what was about to happen began to sink in. Mia started to have vivid dreams about the baby, dreams that left her feeling both exhilarated and terrified. She would wake up in the middle of the night, her heart racing, and Ethan would be there, holding her, reassuring her that everything would be okay.

One night, as they lay in bed, Mia turned to Ethan, her voice barely above a whisper. "Do you think we're really ready for this?"

Ethan looked at her, his eyes filled with love and determination. "I don't think anyone is ever truly ready," he said softly. "But I know that we'll figure it out together. We've come this far, and we've handled everything that's been thrown at us. We'll handle this too."

Mia nodded, tears pricking at the corners of her eyes. "I'm scared, Ethan. I'm scared of the pain, of the unknown, of not being a good mom."

Ethan pulled her close, pressing a kiss to her forehead. "You're going to be an amazing mom, Mia. And I'll be right there with you, every step of the way. We're in this together."

The days leading up to the baby's birth were a whirlwind of last-minute preparations and quiet moments of reflection. Mia and Ethan spent hours talking about their hopes and dreams for their child, imagining what their baby would look like, what kind of personality they would have, and how their lives would change.

They also made sure to carve out time for just the two of them, knowing that once the baby arrived, their lives would be consumed with feedings, diaper changes, and sleepless nights. They went out for dinner, took long walks, and spent lazy Sundays curled up on the couch, savoring the calm before the storm.

And then, one early morning, the time finally came.

Mia woke up to a sharp pain in her abdomen, followed by a slow, steady cramping that grew more intense with each passing minute. She knew, instinctively, that this was it—the beginning of labor. She reached over to wake Ethan, her voice trembling with a mix of fear and excitement.

"Ethan, it's happening. The baby's coming."

Ethan bolted upright, his eyes wide with alarm. "Are you sure? How far apart are the contractions?"

Mia winced as another wave of pain hit her. "They're about ten minutes apart. We should probably call the doctor."

Ethan sprang into action, grabbing the phone and dialing the hospital. He spoke quickly, his voice steady despite the adrenaline coursing through his veins. After getting the necessary instructions, he turned to Mia, his eyes full of determination.

"Okay, let's get you to the hospital."

The drive to the hospital was a blur of sensations—pain, excitement, fear, and a sense of surrealness that made it all feel like a dream. Mia clutched Ethan's hand as the contractions grew stronger, her breath coming in short, sharp gasps.

By the time they arrived at the hospital, Mia was fully in the throes of labor. The nurses whisked her into a room, and the next several hours passed in a haze of pain and exhaustion. Ethan stayed by her side, holding her hand, wiping the sweat from her brow, and whispering words of encouragement.

Mia had never felt anything like this before—the intensity of the contractions, the overwhelming pressure, the sheer physicality of it all. She had always thought of herself as strong, capable of handling anything life threw at her, but this was different. This was raw, primal, and completely out of her control.

But she also felt a deep sense of purpose, a connection to the generations of women who had come before her, who had gone through this same experience and emerged on the other side as mothers. She drew strength from that knowledge, from Ethan's presence, and from the thought of the tiny life that was about to enter the world.

Hours later, after what felt like an eternity, Mia finally heard the sound she had been waiting for— the cry of her newborn baby. The room seemed to blur as the doctor placed the tiny, squirming bundle on her chest, and Mia felt a rush of emotions so powerful that she could barely breathe.

She looked down at the baby, her baby, and the world seemed to shift on its axis. In that moment, nothing else mattered. Not the pain, not the exhaustion, not the fear. All that existed was the small, perfect being in her arms, the culmination of all the changes, all the challenges, and all the love that had brought them to this moment.

Ethan was by her side, his eyes filled with tears as he looked at their child. He reached out to touch the baby's tiny hand, his voice choked with emotion. "Mia, we did it. We're parents."

Mia looked up at him, her heart overflowing with love for the man who had been her partner through it all. "We did it," she whispered, tears streaming down her face. "We're a family."

As they sat there, holding their newborn child, the enormity of what they had accomplished began to sink in. The changes they had navigated, the challenges they had faced, had all led to this—a new beginning, a new chapter in their lives, and a love that would only grow stronger with each passing day.

And in that quiet moment, as the first light of dawn began to filter through the hospital window, Mia and Ethan knew that whatever lay ahead, they would face it together, as a family.

Chapter 6: The First Ultrasound

Mia stood in front of the bathroom mirror, her hand resting on the slight curve of her belly. She still couldn't quite believe it, even after all the morning sickness, the mood swings, and the endless doctor's appointments. Today, she would see the baby for the first time. The thought sent a shiver of excitement down her spine, mingled with a touch of anxiety that she couldn't quite shake.

Ethan was in the bedroom, getting dressed for the appointment. She could hear him humming softly to himself, a habit he'd developed over the past few weeks whenever he was trying to calm his own nerves. Mia smiled to herself, grateful for his presence, his steadiness. They were about to step into a new chapter of their lives together, and she was glad he was by her side.

As they drove to the clinic, the city seemed unusually quiet, as if the world was holding its breath along with them. The autumn leaves drifted down from the trees, covering the sidewalks in a blanket of red and gold. Mia stared out the window, trying to keep her mind from racing. What if something was wrong? What if the ultrasound revealed a problem they weren't prepared for? She knew it was normal to worry, but that didn't make it any easier.

Ethan reached over and took her hand, giving it a reassuring squeeze. "It's going to be okay," he said, as if reading her thoughts.

Mia nodded, though her stomach was still in knots. "I know. I just… I can't help but think of all the things that could go wrong."

"We've come this far," Ethan reminded her. "We're strong, and we're in this together. Whatever happens, we'll face it together."

His words brought her some comfort, and she leaned back in her seat, focusing on the rhythm of his breathing. She loved the way he could ground her, bring her back to the present moment when her mind started to spiral.

When they arrived at the clinic, Mia felt a fresh wave of anxiety wash over her. The waiting room was filled with other expectant couples, some of them looking just as nervous as she felt. She checked in at the front desk, and they took seats by the window, where the morning sun streamed in, casting a warm glow over the room.

Ethan picked up a magazine, flipping through the pages without really looking at them. Mia watched him for a moment, then turned her attention to the other women in the room. Some of them had visible baby bumps, their pregnancies further along than hers. She wondered what they were thinking, whether they were as nervous as she was, or if they had already been through this process and were now simply going through the motions.

After what felt like an eternity, a nurse called Mia's name. She and Ethan followed her down a long corridor to the ultrasound room, their footsteps echoing in the quiet. The room was small and dimly lit, with a large machine taking up most of the space. The nurse gestured for Mia to lie down on the exam table, and she did so, trying to calm the butterflies in her stomach.

Ethan stood beside her, his hand still in hers. The nurse asked a few routine questions as she prepared the equipment, her tone professional yet kind. Mia appreciated the way she moved with quiet efficiency, as if she understood that this was a moment of great importance.

The door opened, and Dr. Patel walked in, her presence bringing a wave of relief to Mia. She had met the doctor a few times before and had always found her to be warm and reassuring. Today, however, Mia was hyperaware of every detail, every nuance, searching for signs that everything would be okay.

"Good morning, Mia, Ethan," Dr. Patel greeted them with a smile. "How are we feeling today?"

"Nervous," Mia admitted, her voice trembling slightly.

"That's completely normal," Dr. Patel assured her. "The first ultrasound is always a big moment. But from everything we've seen so far, there's no reason to worry. Let's take a look and see how things are progressing, shall we?"

Mia nodded, unable to find her voice. Dr. Patel applied a cool gel to her abdomen, and Mia shivered slightly at the sensation. Then, the doctor placed the ultrasound wand on her belly, and the room fell silent as everyone focused on the screen.

For a few moments, there was nothing but a blur of grey and white, the sound of the machine's hum filling the room. Mia held her breath, her heart pounding in her chest. And then, there it was—a tiny, fluttering shape in the center of the screen.

"There's your baby," Dr. Patel said softly, a smile spreading across her face.

Mia's breath caught in her throat. The image on the screen was grainy and indistinct, but there was no mistaking the tiny form nestled within her womb. A rush of emotion surged through her—relief, joy, awe, and an overwhelming sense of love for this little life she had yet to meet.

Ethan stared at the screen, his eyes wide with wonder. "That's our baby," he murmured, his voice thick with emotion.

Mia nodded, tears spilling down her cheeks. She had imagined this moment so many times, but nothing could have prepared her for the reality of it. The baby's heartbeat filled the room, a rapid, steady rhythm that seemed to echo in her chest.

Dr. Patel pointed out different features on the screen—the head, the tiny limbs, the beating heart. "Everything looks great," she said reassuringly. "The baby is developing right on track. You're about twelve weeks along, which lines up perfectly with your last period."

Mia and Ethan exchanged a look of pure relief. Hearing that everything was normal, that their baby was healthy, was like a weight lifting off their shoulders. They had been holding their breath for so long, and now, they could finally exhale.

As the doctor continued to explain what they were seeing, Mia found herself unable to take her eyes off the screen. The baby was so small, so fragile, yet already so full of life. She watched in awe as the little form moved slightly, a tiny flutter of movement that sent a fresh wave of emotion through her.

"This is real," Mia whispered, more to herself than to anyone else. "This is really happening."

Ethan squeezed her hand, his own eyes damp with tears. "Yeah, it is," he said, his voice full of wonder.

Dr. Patel finished the scan and handed Mia a few printed images of the ultrasound. "Here are your first baby pictures," she said with a smile. "You can keep these as a memento."

Mia took the photos with trembling hands, staring down at the black-and-white images. It was surreal to think that this tiny, blurry shape was their child, the baby they had created together. She felt a deep, primal connection to the little life growing inside her, a bond that was both exhilarating and terrifying.

After the ultrasound, Mia and Ethan scheduled a follow-up appointment, then made their way back to the car. The drive home was quiet, both of them lost in their thoughts. Mia kept glancing at the ultrasound photos, her heart swelling with a mixture of love and disbelief.

When they arrived home, Mia placed the ultrasound photos on the coffee table, propping them up against a stack of books. She and Ethan sat on the couch, staring at the images in silence.

"It's so strange," Mia said finally, her voice barely above a whisper. "To think that this little person is inside me, growing every day."

Ethan nodded, his gaze still fixed on the photos. "I know. It's… I don't even have words for it."

Mia leaned her head on his shoulder, feeling the steady rise and fall of his breath. "I'm so glad everything is okay," she said softly. "I've been so worried."

Ethan wrapped an arm around her, pulling her close. "Me too. But the baby is healthy, and that's all that matters."

They sat like that for a long time, basking in the quiet joy of the moment. The ultrasound had made everything feel more real, more tangible. They were no longer just imagining their baby—they had seen it, heard its heartbeat, and connected with it in a way that was impossible to describe.

As the days passed, Mia found herself returning to the ultrasound photos again and again. She carried them with her, tucked into her purse or her journal, taking them out whenever she needed a reminder of the life growing inside her. She showed them to her close friends and family, beaming with pride as they cooed over the tiny form on the screen.

For Mia, the ultrasound was a turning point. It marked the moment when she truly began to see herself as a mother, to embrace the changes happening in her body and her life. She started to think more about the future, about what kind of parent she wanted to be, and about the life she and Ethan were creating together.

Ethan, too, felt a shift in his perspective. Seeing the baby on the ultrasound had made everything more concrete, more immediate. He found himself thinking more about the practical aspects of fatherhood—how to baby-proof the house, what kind of car seat to buy, and how they would manage their finances with a new addition to the family.

But it wasn't just the practicalities that occupied his mind. He also found himself daydreaming about what their baby would be like—whether it would have Mia's eyes or his smile, what their first words would be, what kind of person they would grow up to be. These thoughts filled him with a mixture of excitement and responsibility, a deepening sense of what it meant to be a father.

One evening, a few days after the ultrasound, Mia and Ethan sat on the couch, flipping through a baby name book. They had picked it up on a whim, but now, it felt like an essential part of their journey. The ultrasound had made everything more real, and with that reality came the need to prepare, to plan for the life they were bringing into the world.

"What do you think of Emma for a girl?" Mia asked, tracing her finger down the list of names.

Ethan tilted his head, considering. "I like it. Classic, but still modern. What about Noah for a boy?"

Mia smiled. "I've always liked that name. It's strong, but gentle."

They continued to go through the book, laughing and debating over names, imagining what their child might be like, what kind of life they would lead. It was a moment of connection, of shared dreams and hopes, and it brought them closer together in a way that nothing else could.

The weeks following the ultrasound were a time of quiet anticipation. Mia's belly began to round out more noticeably, and she found herself feeling more connected to the baby with each passing day. She started to feel little flutters, tiny movements that were both thrilling and surreal. Each time she felt the baby move, she would place a hand on her belly, a smile spreading across her face.

Ethan was just as eager to feel the baby's movements. Every evening, he would sit beside Mia on the couch, his hand on her belly, waiting patiently for the slightest sign of life. The first time he felt a kick, his eyes lit up with amazement, and he looked at Mia with a mixture of awe and love.

"That's our baby," he whispered, his voice full of wonder.

Mia nodded, her heart swelling with emotion. "It is," she said softly.

These moments of connection, of feeling the baby move and grow, brought Mia and Ethan closer together. They spent hours talking about the future, about their hopes and dreams for their child. They planned the nursery, picked out baby clothes, and made lists of all the things they would need.

But it wasn't just about the practicalities. It was also about the emotions, the deepening bond between them as they prepared to become parents. They shared their fears and anxieties, their hopes and dreams, and in doing so, they grew stronger together.

As the second trimester progressed, Mia found herself feeling more at ease with her pregnancy. The worries that had plagued her in the beginning began to fade, replaced by a sense of excitement and anticipation. The ultrasound had given her a new perspective, a deeper understanding of the life growing inside her.

She started to embrace the changes in her body, finding joy in the way her belly grew, the way her skin seemed to glow with new life. She began to take better care of herself, eating well, exercising, and taking time to relax. She knew that she was nurturing not just herself, but also her baby, and that thought filled her with a sense of purpose.

Ethan, too, was more involved than ever. He attended every doctor's appointment, read every book he could find on pregnancy and fatherhood, and did everything he could to support Mia. He was there for her through the ups and downs, the mood swings and the cravings, the moments of doubt and the bursts of excitement.

One evening, as they lay in bed, Mia turned to Ethan and said, "I'm so glad we're doing this together. I don't know what I would do without you."

Ethan smiled, brushing a strand of hair from her face. "I feel the same way. We're a team, and we're going to be great parents."

Mia nodded, feeling a deep sense of contentment. She knew that the road ahead wouldn't always be easy, but she also knew that they were in it together, and that made all the difference.

As the weeks passed, the excitement for the next ultrasound grew. They had seen their baby once, and now, they were eager to see how much had changed, how much their little one had grown. The first ultrasound had been a turning point, a moment of realization and connection, and they knew that the next one would be just as meaningful.

When the day finally arrived, Mia and Ethan walked into the clinic with a sense of anticipation that was different from the first time. They were no longer filled with the same kind of nervous anxiety. Instead, they were excited, eager to see their baby again, to witness the progress that had been made.

Dr. Patel greeted them warmly, remembering how emotional their first ultrasound had been. "Are you ready to see your little one again?" she asked with a smile.

Mia and Ethan both nodded, their excitement palpable.

As the ultrasound began, the room filled with the familiar hum of the machine, and the screen flickered to life. This time, the image was clearer, more defined. The baby had grown, and they could see the outline of the head, the arms, the legs. It was a moment of pure joy, a confirmation that their baby was thriving, that everything was progressing as it should.

"There's your baby," Dr. Patel said, pointing out the different features on the screen. "Everything looks perfect."

Mia and Ethan stared at the screen, their hearts filled with love and gratitude. This was their baby, their little miracle, and they were witnessing its growth, its development, right before their eyes.

As they left the clinic, ultrasound photos in hand, Mia felt a deep sense of peace. The journey of pregnancy was filled with so many unknowns, so many ups and downs, but in that moment, she knew that everything was going to be okay. She had Ethan by her side, and together, they were ready to face whatever came their way.

And most importantly, they had their baby, growing stronger every day, a symbol of the love and commitment they shared. The first ultrasound had been a glimpse into the future, a promise of the life they were creating together. It was a moment that would stay with them forever, a reminder of the unexpected joy blossoming in their lives.

Chapter 7: Friendship and Support

As the days turned into weeks, Mia found herself relying more and more on the friendships she had cultivated over the years. The pregnancy had brought about a whirlwind of emotions and changes, and while Ethan was a constant source of support, Mia knew that the journey of motherhood was one she needed to navigate with the help of other women who had been through it, or who were going through it with her.

Mia's closest friend, Lily, had been one of the first people she told about the pregnancy. They had been friends since college, sharing everything from late-night study sessions to heartbreaks and triumphs. When Mia broke the news to her, Lily had squealed with delight, immediately launching into a flurry of questions about how Mia was feeling, how Ethan had reacted, and whether she had started thinking about baby names.

"You're going to be the best mom," Lily had said, her voice full of certainty. "And I'm going to be the best honorary auntie ever."

Mia had laughed, feeling a rush of warmth at Lily's enthusiasm. She knew she could count on her friend to be there every step of the way, offering advice, a listening ear, and plenty of encouragement.

One afternoon, a few weeks after the first ultrasound, Mia and Lily met up for lunch at their favorite café. The weather had turned cooler, and the leaves on the trees had begun to change color, painting the city in shades of amber and gold. They sat by the window, sipping warm tea and catching up on each other's lives.

"How are you feeling?" Lily asked, her eyes full of concern. "Any more morning sickness?"

"Not as much, thankfully," Mia replied, stirring honey into her tea. "But I'm still tired all the time. It's like my body is working overtime to grow this baby."

Lily nodded sympathetically. "That's completely normal. Your body is doing something amazing, so it's no wonder you're exhausted. Just make sure you're getting plenty of rest."

Mia smiled, grateful for Lily's understanding. "I'm trying to. It's just hard sometimes, you know? There's so much to think about, so much to prepare for."

"That's why you've got me," Lily said, reaching across the table to squeeze Mia's hand. "Whatever you need, I'm here. Whether it's helping you shop for baby stuff, listening to you vent, or just keeping you company when you need a break. You're not in this alone."

The words brought tears to Mia's eyes. She hadn't realized just how much she needed to hear them until that moment. The weight of the pregnancy, the responsibility of bringing a new life into the world, had been pressing down on her, and knowing that she had a friend who was willing to share that burden made all the difference.

"Thank you," Mia said, her voice thick with emotion. "I don't know what I'd do without you."

Lily waved her hand dismissively. "You'd be fine. But I'm glad you don't have to find out. We're in this together, okay?"

Mia nodded, a smile breaking through the tears. "Okay."

Their conversation shifted to lighter topics, and soon they were laughing and reminiscing about their college days. But underneath the laughter, Mia felt a deep sense of comfort and security. She knew that no matter what challenges lay ahead, she had friends like Lily who would be there to support her.

As the weeks went by, Mia began to reconnect with other friends as well. Some of them were mothers themselves, while others were still navigating their own paths in life. Regardless of their circumstances, each friendship brought something unique to Mia's journey.

One of these friends was Emily, a woman Mia had met at a prenatal yoga class. Emily was about six months pregnant, and they had struck up a conversation after class one day, bonding over their shared experiences of morning sickness and strange pregnancy cravings.

"I swear, I never thought I'd crave pickles and ice cream at the same time," Emily had said, laughing as she recounted her latest midnight snack. "But here we are."

Mia had laughed along with her, relieved to find someone who understood the bizarre aspects of pregnancy. "It's like our bodies have minds of their own."

From that day on, Mia and Emily became fast friends, meeting up regularly for yoga, walks in the park, or just to chat over a cup of herbal tea. Their conversations ranged from the practical—discussing which baby gear was worth investing in—to the emotional, sharing their hopes and fears about motherhood.

"What scares you the most?" Mia asked one day as they sat on a bench in the park, watching the ducks swim lazily across the pond.

Emily thought for a moment, her brow furrowed in concentration. "I think it's the uncertainty," she said finally. "Not knowing what kind of mother I'll be, or whether I'll be able to handle everything that comes with it. There are so many things we can't control, and that terrifies me."

Mia nodded, understanding all too well. "I feel the same way. It's like, no matter how much we prepare, there's always going to be something unexpected. Something we can't plan for."

"Exactly," Emily agreed. "But I guess that's part of the journey, right? Learning to adapt, to go with the flow."

Mia smiled. "Yeah, I suppose it is."

Their friendship became a source of strength for Mia. They were able to share their vulnerabilities, their uncertainties, and in doing so, they found solace in knowing they weren't alone. Emily's experiences, though different from Mia's in many ways, mirrored her own in the fundamental challenges and joys of pregnancy.

Another important friendship in Mia's life was with her coworker, Sarah. Sarah was a few years older than Mia and had two children of her own. She had been through the ups and downs of pregnancy and motherhood, and her advice was always practical and grounded in experience.

When Mia first told Sarah about the pregnancy, she had received a warm hug and a heartfelt congratulations. "You're going to do great," Sarah had said, her tone full of certainty. "And if you ever need advice, or just someone to talk to, I'm here."

True to her word, Sarah became a mentor of sorts, offering tips on everything from managing work-life balance to dealing with pregnancy-related discomforts.

"Remember to take it easy," Sarah advised one day as they sat in the break room at work. "Don't push yourself too hard. Your body is going through a lot, and you need to give yourself permission to rest."

Mia nodded, appreciating the wisdom in Sarah's words. "It's hard sometimes. I feel like I should be able to do everything I did before, but I'm just so tired all the time."

"That's completely normal," Sarah assured her. "You're growing a whole new person. It's okay to slow down, to ask for help when you need it."

Mia took Sarah's words to heart, learning to be more gentle with herself, to listen to her body and take breaks when necessary. She also found herself leaning on Sarah for advice on the more practical aspects of preparing for the baby.

"What do you think about cloth diapers?" Mia asked one afternoon as they were packing up to leave the office.

Sarah chuckled. "They're great if you're committed, but they can be a lot of work. We tried them with our first, but ended up switching to disposables after a few months. It's really a personal choice, though. You might find that they work well for you."

Mia appreciated Sarah's honesty and her willingness to share her experiences without judgment. It was comforting to know that she didn't have to have all the answers, that she could learn and adapt as she went along.

In addition to her friendships with other women, Mia found support in unexpected places. Her relationship with her mother, which had always been close but sometimes strained, deepened as they bonded over the shared experience of motherhood.

When Mia had first told her mother about the pregnancy, she had been met with a mixture of joy and concern. "Are you sure you're ready for this?" her mother had asked, her voice tinged with worry.

"I think so," Mia had replied, though the truth was that she wasn't entirely sure. But as the weeks passed, and her mother began to share stories of her own pregnancies, Mia found herself growing more confident, more certain that she could handle whatever came her way.

One afternoon, Mia and her mother sat on the porch of the family home, sipping lemonade and reminiscing about the past. The sun was warm, and the scent of blooming flowers filled the air.

"I remember when I was pregnant with you," her mother said, a soft smile on her face. "I was so young, and I didn't know what to expect. But when you were born, everything just fell into place. You were this tiny, perfect little thing, and I knew that I would do anything to protect you, to make sure you had the best life possible."

Mia felt a lump rise in her throat. "Were you scared?"

Her mother nodded. "Terrified. But I think that's just part of being a mother. There's always fear, but there's also so much love, so much joy. And that makes it all worth it."

The conversation left Mia feeling more connected to her mother than ever before. She realized that the fears and uncertainties she was experiencing were natural, that every mother goes through them. And she took comfort in knowing that her mother would be there to guide her, to offer wisdom and support as she navigated the journey ahead.

Mia also found herself leaning on her sister, Kate, who had two children of her own. Kate had always been the more practical, no-nonsense sibling, and her straightforward advice was often just what Mia needed.

"You'll be fine," Kate told her one day as they shopped for baby clothes. "The first few months are tough, but you'll get through it. And once you do, you'll wonder how you ever lived without your little one."

Mia appreciated Kate's confidence in her. It gave her the strength to believe in herself, to trust that she could handle whatever challenges came her way.

As the pregnancy progressed, Mia's circle of support grew even wider. Her friends, family, and coworkers all rallied around her, offering help, advice, and encouragement. She knew that she was incredibly fortunate to have so many people in her life who cared about her, who were there to support her every step of the way.

And through it all, Ethan remained her rock, her constant source of love and strength. They navigated the changes together, leaning on each other, growing closer as they prepared for the arrival of their baby.

Mia knew that the road ahead wouldn't always be easy, but with the support of the people she loved, she felt ready to face whatever came her way. The friendships and connections she had built over the years were more important than ever, providing her with the strength and confidence she needed as she embarked on the journey of motherhood.

As she looked around at the people in her life, Mia felt a deep sense of gratitude. The unexpected joy blossoming within her wasn't just about the baby she was carrying; it was also about the love and support that surrounded her, the friendships that had grown stronger, and the new connections she was forming.

In that moment, Mia knew that she wasn't alone. She had a community of people who cared about her, who would be there to support her every step of the way. And with that knowledge, she felt ready to embrace the journey ahead, to welcome the changes, and to face the future with hope and confidence.

Chapter 8: Career Crossroads

As Mia's pregnancy progressed, she found herself at a crossroads, both personally and professionally. The excitement of the baby's arrival was tempered by the realities of balancing work with the demands of impending motherhood. Her career, which had always been a source of pride and fulfillment, was now intertwined with a new set of challenges and decisions.

Mia had always been dedicated to her job as a marketing coordinator at a fast-paced tech company. She enjoyed the creative aspects of her work, the camaraderie with her colleagues, and the sense of accomplishment that came with each successful campaign. But as the months passed and her pregnancy became more apparent, she began to grapple with the impact it would have on her career.

One crisp autumn morning, Mia sat at her desk, surrounded by the familiar hum of office activity. The leaves outside the window had turned brilliant shades of orange and red, a vivid reminder of the changing seasons and the changes in her own life. She found herself staring at her computer screen, feeling a pang of anxiety as she thought about the months ahead.

Her supervisor, Laura, had been supportive of her pregnancy, but as her due date approached, Mia knew she needed to have a conversation about her maternity leave and her plans for returning to work. She wanted to ensure that her transition out of the office and back in afterward would be as smooth as possible, but she wasn't sure how to approach the topic.

"Hey, Mia," Laura said, appearing at her desk with a friendly smile. "Got a minute to chat?"

Mia looked up, trying to hide her nerves. "Sure, Laura. What's up?"

Laura gestured for Mia to follow her to a nearby conference room. Once inside, she closed the door and took a seat across from Mia. "I just wanted to touch base with you about your maternity leave. I know you're getting close to your due date, and I wanted to make sure we're all set for when you're ready to take time off."

Mia nodded, her heart racing. "Yes, I've been meaning to discuss that. I want to make sure everything is in place before I go on leave."

Laura smiled reassuringly. "Of course. We've been planning for your absence and making arrangements to cover your responsibilities. We'll work with you to ensure a smooth handover. Do you have any specific concerns or questions?"

Mia took a deep breath, feeling a mixture of relief and anxiety. "I guess my main concern is how things will work when I return. I want to make sure I'm able to transition back into my role without too much disruption."

Laura's expression softened. "We'll be flexible with your return. We can discuss options for a phased return if that's something you'd be interested in. And of course, if you need any adjustments or accommodations, just let us know."

Mia appreciated Laura's understanding. "That sounds good. I just want to be sure that everything is set up so that I don't have to worry too much about work while I'm on leave."

Laura nodded. "We'll make sure everything is taken care of. And if you have any concerns or need anything, just reach out."

The conversation left Mia feeling more at ease, but she still had lingering doubts about how she would manage the transition back to work. The thought of juggling her career with the demands of a newborn was daunting, and she wondered if it was possible to find a balance that worked for both her and her family.

In the days that followed, Mia found herself contemplating her career more deeply. She had always envisioned herself climbing the corporate ladder, but now she was questioning whether that path was still right for her. The idea of returning to work full-time after maternity leave felt overwhelming, and she wondered if there were alternative options that might better suit her new life as a mother.

One evening, after a particularly long day at the office, Mia sat down with Ethan to discuss her thoughts. They had just finished dinner, and the two of them were curled up on the couch, the soft glow of the lamp casting a warm light over the room.

"I've been thinking a lot about work lately," Mia began, her voice tinged with uncertainty. "And I'm not sure what I want to do after the baby arrives."

Ethan looked at her with concern. "What's on your mind?"

Mia took a deep breath. "I love my job, but I'm worried about how I'll manage everything once the baby is here. I'm thinking about whether it might be better to look for something part-time, or maybe even take a break from my career for a while."

Ethan nodded, listening intently. "I understand. It's a big adjustment, and it's natural to want to rethink things. Have you talked to your boss about these concerns?"

"I did," Mia said, nodding. "Laura was very supportive, but I'm still feeling unsure. I guess I'm just worried about finding the right balance."

Ethan reached over and took her hand. "Whatever you decide, I'm here to support you. We can figure this out together. Maybe we can look into some options and see what might work best for us."

Mia felt a surge of gratitude for Ethan's support. "Thanks. I just want to make sure I'm making the right decision for our family."

Over the next few weeks, Mia began to explore her options. She reached out to other working mothers, seeking their advice on balancing career and family. She also looked into part-time work opportunities and flexible work arrangements, hoping to find a solution that would allow her to continue her career while also being present for her baby.

One afternoon, she met with a former colleague who had transitioned to part-time work after having children. They sat at a cozy café, sipping coffee and discussing the pros and cons of part-time employment.

"It's definitely a balancing act," her colleague said, her tone thoughtful. "But it's also been great to have more time with my kids. I've been able to stay connected with my career while also being more present at home."

Mia listened carefully, weighing the possibilities. "I think I'd like to explore part-time options. I want to stay involved with my work, but I also want to be there for my baby."

Her colleague nodded in agreement. "It's worth discussing with your employer. Many companies are open to flexible arrangements, especially for new parents."

Encouraged by the conversation, Mia began to put together a plan for her career. She crafted a proposal for a part-time or flexible work arrangement and scheduled a meeting with Laura to discuss it. She wanted to present a well-thought-out plan that would address her concerns while also demonstrating her commitment to her role.

The meeting with Laura went smoothly. Mia explained her desire to transition to part-time work and outlined how she planned to manage her responsibilities. Laura was supportive and open to the idea, and together they worked on a plan that would allow Mia to maintain her connection with the company while also having more time for her family.

"Your proposal makes a lot of sense," Laura said, reviewing the plan. "I think this could work well for both you and the team. We'll need to make some adjustments, but I'm confident we can find a solution that works."

Mia felt a sense of relief and accomplishment. The plan wasn't perfect, but it was a step in the right direction, and it gave her hope that she could find a way to balance her career and family life.

As the due date approached, Mia continued to prepare for the arrival of her baby while also wrapping up her work responsibilities. She worked closely with her team to ensure that everything was in place for her maternity leave, and she took comfort in knowing that she had a supportive work environment waiting for her return.

The decision to transition to part-time work was a significant one, and it wasn't without its challenges. But Mia felt confident in her choice and grateful for the support she had received from her employer, her friends, and her family.

As she looked forward to the arrival of her baby, Mia felt a renewed sense of purpose. She knew that the road ahead would be filled with both joys and challenges, but she was ready to embrace it all. With Ethan by her side and a supportive network of friends and colleagues, she felt prepared to navigate the career crossroads and create a new balance in her life.

In the end, Mia realized that the key to finding fulfillment was not about choosing between career and family, but about creating a life that embraced both. She was excited to start this new chapter and to see where the journey would take her, knowing that she had the strength and support to face whatever came her way.

Chapter 9: The Father's Journey

As Mia's pregnancy advanced, Ethan found himself on a deeply personal journey, exploring the nuances of fatherhood and the impact it would have on his life. While he had been supportive from the start, the reality of becoming a father brought forth a whirlwind of emotions and reflections that demanded his full attention.

Ethan had always prided himself on his problem-solving skills and his ability to manage high-pressure situations at work. As a project manager, he thrived on planning, strategizing, and executing complex projects. But the impending arrival of his child introduced an entirely new dimension of uncertainty and responsibility that he hadn't anticipated.

The early days after Mia's announcement were filled with a mixture of elation and anxiety for Ethan. He was thrilled about becoming a father but also overwhelmed by the practical implications of this new role. Balancing his demanding job with the preparations for the baby felt like walking a tightrope.

One of Ethan's first challenges was to reconcile his career ambitions with the reality of impending fatherhood. He had always envisioned climbing the corporate ladder, but the prospect of taking paternity leave and adjusting his work hours made him question his long-term career goals. Ethan wanted to be present for Mia and their baby, but he also wanted to maintain his professional identity and provide for his family.

Ethan's introspection led him to seek advice from colleagues and friends who had navigated similar transitions. During a lunch break, he met with Mark, a friend who had recently become a father. Mark's stories of sleepless nights and the challenges of balancing work and parenting resonated with Ethan.

"It's a balancing act," Mark said, leaning back in his chair with a thoughtful expression. "You'll find that your priorities shift, and it's okay to reevaluate your goals. The key is to be present and flexible."

Ethan nodded, absorbing the wisdom in Mark's words. "I want to be there for Mia and the baby, but I also don't want to jeopardize my career. It's a tough choice."

Mark offered a reassuring smile. "It's about finding a balance that works for you and your family. Communicate with your employer, explore flexible options, and remember that it's okay to ask for help."

Inspired by the conversation, Ethan began to explore ways to make his transition into fatherhood smoother. He had a candid discussion with his manager about his upcoming paternity leave and the possibility of flexible work arrangements. His manager was understanding and supportive, and together they devised a plan that would allow Ethan to be present for Mia and their baby while continuing to contribute to his team.

The process of preparing for the baby's arrival also brought Ethan closer to Mia. He took an active role in attending prenatal appointments, eagerly watching the ultrasound scans and participating in discussions about baby names and nursery décor. Each milestone in the pregnancy deepened his connection to the experience and reinforced his commitment to being an engaged father.

One evening, as Mia and Ethan worked together to assemble the nursery furniture, they found themselves in a reflective mood. Mia was carefully arranging baby clothes in the dresser while Ethan struggled to assemble a crib. Frustration tinged his voice as he tried to fit the pieces together.

"Need some help?" Mia asked, her tone both playful and encouraging.

Ethan looked up, a sheepish grin on his face. "I think I might need more than just help. I might need a miracle."

Mia laughed softly and walked over to lend a hand. As they worked side by side, Ethan couldn't help but marvel at the progress they were making. The nursery was taking shape, and the reality of their impending parenthood was becoming more tangible.

"I've been thinking a lot about what kind of father I want to be," Ethan said, his voice thoughtful. "I want to be there for you and our baby, but I also want to make sure I'm doing my part to support our family."

Mia looked up from the dresser, her eyes filled with warmth. "You're already doing so much. Being here with me, helping with the preparations—it means a lot. I know you'll be a great father."

Ethan felt a swell of gratitude and determination. "I hope so. I just want to make sure I'm doing everything I can to support you and be there for our baby."

As the due date approached, Ethan found himself balancing anticipation with nervousness. He had read parenting books, attended classes with Mia, and made practical preparations, but the unknowns of parenthood still loomed large. He often lay awake at night, imagining the challenges and joys that lay ahead.

In the final weeks of the pregnancy, Ethan took time off work to focus on supporting Mia and preparing for the baby's arrival. He attended childbirth classes with her, learned about newborn care, and made sure that everything was in place for the baby's homecoming. His dedication to being involved was evident in every action, from assembling furniture to organizing supplies.

The night of Mia's labor arrived with a mix of excitement and anxiety. Ethan was by her side every step of the way, offering encouragement and support. The experience was both exhilarating and overwhelming, and Ethan found himself in awe of Mia's strength and resilience.

When their baby finally arrived, Ethan's heart swelled with emotion. The moment he held their child for the first time was a profound and transformative experience. He felt an overwhelming sense of love and responsibility, knowing that he was now part of a new chapter in their lives.

As they settled into their new routine as parents, Ethan continued to navigate the challenges of balancing work and family life. He worked with his employer to establish a flexible work arrangement that allowed him to spend quality time with his family while continuing to contribute professionally.

The journey of fatherhood was not without its difficulties, but Ethan embraced each challenge with determination and love. He found joy in the small moments—changing diapers, soothing a fussy baby, and sharing late-night feedings with Mia. Each experience reinforced his commitment to being a supportive and involved father.

In the months that followed, Ethan's role as a father became an integral part of his identity. He continued to balance his career with his responsibilities at home, finding fulfillment in both aspects of his life. The support of Mia, their baby, and their extended family helped him navigate the complexities of parenthood with resilience and grace.

Ethan's journey as a father was a testament to his growth and dedication. He had faced his fears, embraced his new role, and found a way to harmonize his career aspirations with the joys and responsibilities of parenthood. Through it all, he remained steadfast in his commitment to his family, ready to embrace each new challenge and cherish every moment of this transformative journey.

Chapter 10: Family Tensions

As Mia and Ethan prepared for the arrival of their baby, they found themselves navigating not only the challenges of impending parenthood but also the complexities of family dynamics. While their immediate families were generally supportive, underlying tensions and differing expectations began to surface, adding a layer of stress to their journey.

The initial excitement of sharing the news of Mia's pregnancy had been met with a flurry of congratulatory messages and enthusiastic responses. However, as the reality of the impending arrival set in, the interactions with family members began to reveal deeper issues that Mia and Ethan had to address.

One evening, as Mia and Ethan settled in for dinner at Mia's parents' house, the conversation took a turn toward baby preparations. Mia's mother, Joan, was bustling around the kitchen, arranging plates and serving dishes with her usual efficiency. Her father, Robert, was seated at the table, flipping through a magazine and occasionally joining in the conversation.

"So, have you decided on a name yet?" Joan asked, her tone light but with an undercurrent of curiosity.

Mia and Ethan exchanged a glance. "We're still considering a few options," Mia replied, trying to keep the conversation casual.

Joan nodded, but Robert looked up from his magazine with a thoughtful expression. "You know, we had some strong opinions on names when you were born. It's important to choose something meaningful."

Mia felt a pang of discomfort. "We appreciate your input, but we're trying to find a name that feels right for us."

The conversation quickly shifted to other topics, but the underlying tension lingered. Joan's well-meaning but persistent suggestions about baby names and parenting choices began to feel overwhelming to Mia. She wanted to honor her parents' opinions but also needed to assert her own choices as an expectant mother.

In the weeks that followed, similar tensions arose with Ethan's family. They had been supportive initially, but as the due date approached, they began to express their own concerns and expectations. Ethan's mother, Linda, had been particularly vocal about her ideas for baby care and parenting practices.

One Sunday afternoon, Ethan and Mia visited Linda's house for lunch. The conversation turned to the baby's upcoming arrival, and Linda eagerly shared her advice on everything from feeding schedules to sleep training.

"You know, when you were a baby, we did things a certain way, and it worked out just fine," Linda said, her tone firm. "I think you should consider doing it like we did."

Ethan, trying to balance his desire to respect his mother's input with his commitment to supporting Mia's choices, found himself in a difficult position. "We're looking into various methods and making decisions based on what works best for us."

Linda's expression tightened, and a momentary silence followed. "Well, just remember that there's a lot of experience and wisdom in what we did."

The conversation left Ethan feeling conflicted. He wanted to honor his mother's experience while also asserting his and Mia's independence as new parents. He understood that the advice came from a place of love, but the pressure to conform to traditional practices was causing strain.

As the days went by, the family tensions continued to simmer. Mia and Ethan found themselves caught between their own desires and the expectations of their families. They knew they needed to address these issues but were unsure of how to approach the conversations without causing further friction.

One evening, after a particularly tense discussion with their families, Mia and Ethan sat down together to process their feelings. They were both exhausted from the constant juggling of differing opinions and the pressure to meet everyone's expectations.

"I feel like we're caught in the middle," Mia said, her voice tinged with frustration. "I want to make choices that are right for us, but it's hard when everyone has their own ideas about how things should be."

Ethan sighed, nodding in agreement. "It's challenging to balance our own preferences with the expectations of our families. I don't want to hurt anyone's feelings, but I also want us to feel confident in our decisions."

Mia reached out and took Ethan's hand. "We need to find a way to navigate this together. We have to be firm about our choices and communicate our boundaries clearly."

Ethan squeezed her hand, feeling a renewed sense of determination. "You're right. We need to stand up for ourselves and make decisions that feel right for us. We can't let the pressure from our families dictate everything."

With a plan in mind, Mia and Ethan decided to have open and honest conversations with their families. They wanted to express their gratitude for the support and advice but also make it clear that they needed space to make their own decisions as parents.

One Saturday afternoon, they invited both sets of parents over for a family discussion. The atmosphere was tense but filled with a sense of purpose as Mia and Ethan prepared to address the issues.

As everyone gathered in the living room, Mia took a deep breath and began. "We're really grateful for all the support and advice we've received from both of you. It means a lot to us that you care about our growing family."

Joan and Linda exchanged glances, their expressions softening. "We just want what's best for you and the baby," Joan said, her voice gentle.

Mia nodded. "We understand that, and we appreciate your input. However, we need to make decisions that feel right for us as parents. We're trying to navigate this new chapter in our own way, and it's important to us that we have the freedom to do that."

Ethan added, "We hope you can understand our perspective. We value your advice, but we also need to establish our own approach to parenting."

The conversation was difficult but productive. Joan and Linda listened and acknowledged Mia and Ethan's perspective, though the adjustment was not without its challenges. Both sets of parents had their own emotions and reactions to process, but the open dialogue helped to clarify boundaries and expectations.

As the weeks went by, the family tensions began to ease. While there were still occasional moments of disagreement, Mia and Ethan felt more confident in their ability to navigate the complexities of their family dynamics. They continued to communicate openly and assertively, finding a balance between honoring their families' input and staying true to their own choices.

The arrival of their baby marked a new chapter in their lives, and with it came a renewed sense of unity and purpose. Mia and Ethan had faced the challenges of family tensions head-on and emerged with a stronger understanding of their own needs and boundaries.

In the end, the journey through family tensions was a reminder of the importance of clear communication, mutual respect, and the courage to stand firm in one's decisions. Mia and Ethan's experience taught them that navigating the complexities of family dynamics was an ongoing process, one that required patience, empathy, and a shared commitment to creating a loving and supportive environment for their growing family.

Chapter 11: Preparations

As Mia and Ethan approached the final stretch of their pregnancy journey, the anticipation of their baby's arrival filled their days with both excitement and urgency. With the due date drawing near, the couple found themselves immersed in a whirlwind of preparations, each task bringing them closer to the moment they had been eagerly awaiting.

The nursery, once a blank canvas, was now beginning to take shape. Mia and Ethan had spent countless hours selecting furniture, choosing colors, and arranging the space to create a welcoming environment for their baby. The walls were painted a soft, soothing shade of pastel, and the crib, lovingly assembled by Ethan, stood as the centerpiece of the room. A mobile adorned with whimsical animals hung above the crib, gently swaying with the breeze from the open window.

One Saturday morning, Mia and Ethan decided to tackle the final touches on the nursery. Mia was busy organizing baby clothes and accessories, folding tiny onesies and arranging them neatly in drawers. Ethan was assembling a changing table, carefully following the instructions and making sure each piece was securely fastened.

"I can't believe how quickly this room has come together," Mia said, looking around with a sense of satisfaction. "It feels so real now."

Ethan glanced up from his work, a smile on his face. "It really does. I'm excited to see it all come together."

The preparations extended beyond the nursery. Mia and Ethan also focused on practical tasks such as stocking up on baby supplies and setting up a support system for when the baby arrived. They spent weekends purchasing essentials like diapers, wipes, and baby care products, carefully choosing items that they felt were best for their new arrival.

One afternoon, they visited a local baby store to pick up a few last-minute items. The aisles were filled with an array of products, from adorable baby clothes to high-tech gadgets. Mia and Ethan navigated the store, making selections based on their preferences and budget.

"Do we really need a fancy bottle warmer?" Ethan asked, holding up a sleek appliance with various settings.

Mia considered the question, her brow furrowed in thought. "It might be convenient, especially during late-night feedings. But we should weigh whether it's something we'll use often."

They decided to go with a more basic model and added it to their cart. As they continued shopping, they joked and laughed, finding moments of lightness amidst the flurry of tasks.

In addition to practical preparations, Mia and Ethan also focused on creating a birthing plan. They had discussed their preferences for labor and delivery and wanted to ensure that they were both prepared for the experience. They attended childbirth classes together, learning about different stages of labor, pain management options, and the roles of various support people.

One evening, they sat down to draft their birthing plan. Mia held a notepad, jotting down their preferences while Ethan reviewed a list of options they had discussed in class.

"I'd like to have a calm and supportive environment," Mia said, her voice steady. "I'd prefer to avoid unnecessary interventions if possible."

Ethan nodded in agreement. "And I'd like to be as involved as possible, offering support and encouragement throughout the process. I want to make sure we're both comfortable and informed."

They completed the birthing plan and made copies to share with their healthcare provider and the hospital staff. The process of creating the plan brought them closer and helped them feel more in control of their upcoming experience.

As the days passed, Mia and Ethan also turned their attention to organizing their home for the arrival of the baby. They made sure to have everything in place, from setting up a safe sleeping area to preparing a designated space for baby care essentials. They created a checklist of tasks and worked through it systematically, ensuring that no detail was overlooked.

One evening, they sat together in the living room, reviewing their checklist. The room was filled with the soft glow of a lamp, and the air was tinged with a sense of accomplishment.

"We're almost there," Ethan said, his voice filled with relief. "It feels good to see everything coming together."

Mia smiled, resting her hand on her round belly. "It really does. I'm so grateful for all the support we've received and the hard work we've put in."

They took a moment to reflect on the journey that had brought them to this point. The preparations for their baby's arrival had been both exhilarating and challenging, but they had faced each task with determination and care. The process had strengthened their bond and deepened their appreciation for each other.

As the due date approached, Mia and Ethan found themselves eagerly anticipating the arrival of their baby. They felt ready, both practically and emotionally, for the next chapter in their lives. The nursery was complete, the supplies were stocked, and their birthing plan was in place.

The final days before the baby's arrival were filled with a mix of excitement and nervous energy. Mia and Ethan spent their time reviewing their plans, making last-minute adjustments, and savoring the final moments of their time as a couple before becoming parents.

On one of these final days, Mia and Ethan decided to take a break from their preparations and enjoy a quiet evening together. They went for a walk in the park, enjoying the fresh air and the beauty of nature. As they strolled hand in hand, they reflected on the journey they had been on and the changes that lay ahead.

"I'm so grateful for everything we've accomplished together," Mia said, her voice filled with emotion. "I know we've faced challenges, but we've also made so many wonderful memories."

Ethan squeezed her hand gently. "I feel the same way. We've worked hard to get to this point, and I'm excited for what's to come."

The walk ended with a peaceful moment under the stars, and the couple returned home feeling content and ready for the next chapter. The preparations had been thorough and thoughtful, and they were eager to welcome their baby into the world.

As the due date approached, Mia and Ethan's home was filled with a sense of anticipation and readiness. They had prepared meticulously and were now ready to embrace the joys and challenges of parenthood. The journey had been a testament to their love, dedication, and commitment to creating a nurturing environment for their growing family.

Chapter 12: The Baby Shower

The anticipation of the baby's arrival was building to a crescendo as Mia's baby shower approached. It was a milestone moment for Mia and Ethan, an opportunity to celebrate with family and friends and to prepare for the final stretch before the baby's arrival. The planning for the shower had been a collaborative effort, involving both families and close friends, and Mia felt a mix of excitement and nerves as the big day drew near.

The baby shower was set to take place at Mia's parents' house, which had been transformed into a vibrant and festive venue. Joan had taken charge of the decorations, transforming the living room with pastel balloons, streamers, and a banner that read "Welcome Baby!" The room was adorned with an array of floral arrangements and a table filled with a variety of delicious foods and treats.

As the guests began to arrive, Mia and Ethan greeted them with warm smiles. The atmosphere was filled with the buzz of conversation and laughter, and Mia felt a wave of gratitude for the support and love surrounding them.

Mia's best friend, Emily, had taken on the role of hostess, ensuring that everything ran smoothly.

She had organized a series of fun games and activities, including a diaper raffle, a baby trivia quiz, and a "guess the baby food" challenge. The games were met with enthusiastic participation, and the room was filled with laughter and friendly competition.

Mia's family and friends gathered around the gift table, excitedly presenting their carefully chosen presents. As Mia opened each gift, she was touched by the thoughtfulness and generosity of her loved ones. There were onesies, blankets, toys, and books, each item a symbol of the support and love that surrounded her.

One of the most touching moments of the shower was when Mia's grandmother, Eleanor, presented her with a hand-knitted blanket. Eleanor had spent countless hours creating the blanket, and the care and effort she had put into it were evident in every stitch.

"This is beautiful, Grandma," Mia said, her voice choked with emotion as she held the blanket close. "Thank you so much."

Eleanor smiled, her eyes twinkling with warmth. "I wanted to make something special for my great-grandchild. I hope it brings you comfort and joy."

The baby shower was also a time for Mia and Ethan to reflect on the journey that had brought them to this point. As they mingled with their guests and enjoyed the festivities, they felt a deep sense of appreciation for the community of people who had supported them throughout the pregnancy.

During the shower, Ethan took a moment to connect with some of the men who were attending. He gathered with a few friends and family members, discussing their own experiences and offering advice on fatherhood. The camaraderie and shared experiences provided Ethan with a sense of reassurance and solidarity as he prepared for his new role.

One of Ethan's friends, David, who was already a father of two, shared his own insights. "It's a wild ride, but it's worth every moment. Just remember to be patient and enjoy the little things."

Ethan nodded, taking in David's advice. "Thanks for the encouragement. It's reassuring to hear from someone who's been through it."

As the afternoon progressed, Mia and Ethan found themselves surrounded by a sea of well-wishers, each offering their own unique words of encouragement and advice. The baby shower was a celebration of not only the impending arrival of their baby but also the love and support that had been a constant source of strength throughout the pregnancy.

The highlight of the shower was the time spent sharing stories and experiences with loved ones. Mia's friends and family shared their own memories of parenting, offering a mix of humor, wisdom, and heartfelt advice. The conversations ranged from tales of sleepless nights to tips on baby care, creating an atmosphere of camaraderie and shared experience.

As the baby shower drew to a close, Mia and Ethan felt a profound sense of gratitude. They had been surrounded by people who cared deeply for them and their growing family, and the support they received was both heartwarming and uplifting.

Joan and Emily coordinated a group photo with all the guests, capturing the joyous moment. Mia and Ethan stood at the center, surrounded by their loved ones, each person beaming with happiness and anticipation for the new arrival.

As the guests began to depart, Mia and Ethan took a moment to reflect on the day's events. They stood together in the living room, surrounded by the remnants of the celebration and the pile of gifts.

"That was amazing," Mia said, her eyes shining with emotion. "I'm so grateful for everyone who came and for all the love and support we've received."

Ethan wrapped his arm around her, his smile reflecting the same sense of gratitude. "It really was. I feel so lucky to have such a wonderful support system. It makes me even more excited to welcome our baby into this world."

With the baby shower behind them, Mia and Ethan turned their attention to the final preparations for their baby's arrival. The shower had been a reminder of the strength of their support network and the joy that awaited them in the coming weeks.

As they began to organize the gifts and make final adjustments to the nursery, Mia and Ethan felt a renewed sense of readiness and anticipation. The baby shower had been a celebration of love and support, and it had prepared them for the next chapter in their lives.

With hearts full of gratitude and excitement, Mia and Ethan embraced the final days before their baby's arrival, ready to welcome their child into a world filled with love, joy, and the unwavering support of their family and friends.

Chapter 13: The Final Stretch

As the due date loomed on the horizon, Mia and Ethan found themselves in the midst of the final stretch of their pregnancy journey. The last few weeks before the baby's arrival were filled with a blend of anticipation, preparation, and a touch of nervousness. The countdown was on, and every day brought them closer to meeting their little one.

Mia's days were marked by a growing sense of both excitement and impatience. The physical discomforts of late pregnancy were becoming more pronounced, with swelling feet, a heavy belly, and frequent trips to the bathroom. Despite these challenges, Mia remained upbeat and focused on the positive aspects of the final stretch.

One evening, as Mia sat on the couch with her feet propped up, Ethan joined her with a cup of herbal tea. He handed it to her with a gentle smile, knowing how much she appreciated these small gestures of support.

"How are you feeling?" Ethan asked, settling beside her.

Mia took a sip of the tea and sighed contentedly. "I'm definitely feeling the weight of it all, but I'm excited. It's hard to believe we're so close."

Ethan nodded, his hand resting on her belly. "It's incredible. I can't wait to finally meet our baby."

The final stretch was also a time for Mia and Ethan to focus on any last-minute preparations. They reviewed their birthing plan, double-checked their hospital bag, and made sure everything was in order. They had also scheduled their final prenatal appointments and were in regular contact with their healthcare provider.

At one of their final appointments, Mia and Ethan met with Dr. Simmons, their obstetrician. The visit was routine but important as they approached the end of the pregnancy.

"Everything looks great," Dr. Simmons said, reviewing Mia's charts. "The baby is in a good position, and there are no concerns at this point. Just keep an eye out for any signs of labor and don't hesitate to call us if you have any questions."

Mia and Ethan left the appointment feeling reassured but also aware of the growing anticipation. They had been counting down the days and had reached the point where they were ready for the baby to arrive.

In the evenings, Mia and Ethan would take quiet walks together, enjoying the calm before the impending arrival. The walks were a time for them to connect, share their thoughts, and reflect on the journey they had been on.

"I've been thinking about how much our lives are going to change," Mia said during one of their walks. "It's exciting but also a little overwhelming."

Ethan squeezed her hand gently. "I know what you mean. It's a big transition, but we're going to handle it together. We've got this."

As the due date approached, Mia's thoughts were often filled with a mix of emotions. She experienced moments of excitement, anxiety, and a deep sense of anticipation. The physical discomforts of late pregnancy were challenging, but she tried to focus on the positive aspects of this final stretch.

Mia's family and friends continued to offer their support and encouragement. Joan, in particular, checked in regularly, offering to help with anything Mia might need. The gestures of kindness and support provided a comforting reminder of the community surrounding them.

One afternoon, Mia and Ethan spent time organizing their home, ensuring everything was in place for the baby's arrival. They made final adjustments to the nursery, arranging the baby's clothes, and setting up the essentials.

As they worked together, Ethan glanced over at Mia, his expression filled with admiration. "You've done an amazing job preparing for this baby. I'm so proud of you."

Mia smiled, feeling a sense of accomplishment. "Thank you. I'm excited, and I'm grateful for everything we've done together. It's been a lot of work, but it's all worth it."

The final days before the baby's arrival were a mix of mundane tasks and moments of reflection. Mia and Ethan spent time enjoying each other's company, preparing for the changes ahead, and savoring the calm before the storm.

One evening, they decided to have a quiet dinner at home, focusing on enjoying each other's company and relaxing before the baby arrived. They prepared a simple meal, setting the table with candles and soft music in the background.

As they sat down to eat, Ethan looked across the table at Mia, his eyes filled with warmth. "I've been thinking about how lucky we are to have each other. This journey has brought us even closer."

Mia reached across the table, taking Ethan's hand. "I feel the same way. It's been an incredible journey, and I'm so grateful to have you by my side."

The dinner was a peaceful and intimate moment, a reminder of the love and support that had carried them through the pregnancy. As they finished their meal, Mia and Ethan felt a renewed sense of readiness and excitement for the arrival of their baby.

In the final days, Mia found herself reflecting on the journey that had brought her to this point. She thought about the early days of the pregnancy, the challenges they had faced, and the support they had received from their loved ones. The experience had been transformative, and she felt a deep sense of gratitude for the path that had led her to this moment.

One night, as Mia and Ethan lay in bed, they talked about their hopes and dreams for their baby. The conversation was filled with love and anticipation as they imagined their future together as a family.

"I hope our baby knows how much we love them," Mia said, her voice soft.

Ethan smiled, brushing a strand of hair from her face. "They will. We're going to give them all the love and support they need."

As the due date approached, Mia and Ethan were ready to embrace the final stretch of their journey. They had prepared thoughtfully, supported each other through the ups and downs, and were eagerly anticipating the moment when they would finally meet their baby.

The final days were a time of quiet anticipation, a chance for Mia and Ethan to savor the calm before the arrival of their little one. With hearts full of hope and excitement, they looked forward to the next chapter in their lives, ready to welcome their baby with open arms and loving hearts.

Chapter 14: Labor and Delivery

The night sky was filled with a blanket of stars as Mia and Ethan prepared for bed. The final stretch of Mia's pregnancy had been a time of anticipation and excitement, and tonight was no different. As they settled into their routine, little did they know that their lives were about to change in a profound and unforgettable way.

Mia had been feeling occasional contractions throughout the day, but they were sporadic and not particularly intense. Ethan, ever attentive, kept a close eye on Mia's comfort and well-being. They had discussed the signs of labor extensively and were both prepared for whatever might come.

Just after midnight, Mia woke with a jolt, her breath coming in short, sharp bursts. A contraction had taken her by surprise, and it was stronger than any she had experienced before. She shifted in bed, trying to find a comfortable position, but the discomfort persisted.

"Mia, are you okay?" Ethan's voice was laced with concern as he noticed her restlessness.

"I'm having a contraction," Mia replied, her voice strained. "It's definitely stronger than before."

Ethan immediately sprang into action. He checked the time and began timing the contractions, as they had learned in their prenatal classes. The contractions were coming at regular intervals, and they seemed to be intensifying.

"We should call the hospital," Ethan said, his tone serious. "This might be it."

Mia nodded, trying to stay calm. Ethan made the call, and after speaking with the nurse on duty, they were advised to come in to be evaluated. As

Ethan gathered their hospital bag and prepared the car, Mia took deep breaths, focusing on managing the contractions.

The drive to the hospital was a blur of nerves and excitement. The streets were quiet, and the car ride felt both surreal and exhilarating. Mia and Ethan held hands, exchanging reassuring glances as they navigated the journey.

Upon arriving at the hospital, they were greeted by the staff and guided to the labor and delivery unit. Mia was wheeled to a private room, and the medical team quickly assessed her condition. The nurses were warm and professional, helping Mia to settle into the bed and monitoring her vital signs.

Dr. Simmons, their obstetrician, arrived shortly thereafter. She conducted an examination and confirmed that Mia was indeed in active labor. The news brought a wave of relief and excitement to both Mia and Ethan.

"Everything is progressing well," Dr. Simmons said with a reassuring smile. "We'll monitor you closely and support you through the process."

Mia's contractions continued to build in intensity, and she focused on her breathing techniques to manage the pain. Ethan was by her side, providing comfort and encouragement. He offered sips of water, gently massaged her back, and held her hand through each contraction.

As the hours passed, Mia's labor progressed. The contractions became more frequent and intense, and she relied on Ethan and the medical team for support. The room was filled with a sense of anticipation, as Mia and Ethan prepared for the final stages of labor.

The support of the medical team was invaluable. The nurses provided guidance on various labor positions and techniques to ease Mia's discomfort. They helped her change positions, encouraged her to use a birthing ball, and offered continuous reassurance.

Despite the intensity of the labor, Mia found strength in Ethan's presence. His steady hand, soothing voice, and unwavering support provided a sense of calm amidst the chaos of the experience.

As Mia approached the pushing stage, the room transformed into a hive of activity. Dr. Simmons prepared for delivery, and the nursing staff readied the necessary equipment. Mia was given instructions on how to push effectively, and the process began.

The pushing stage was a challenging yet empowering experience for Mia. She focused on her breathing and followed the guidance of Dr. Simmons and the nurses. Ethan remained by her side, offering words of encouragement and support.

With each push, Mia could feel progress being made. The energy in the room was palpable, and the anticipation was almost overwhelming. Ethan's eyes were filled with pride and awe as he witnessed Mia's strength and determination.

After what felt like an eternity, but was in reality a matter of hours, Mia felt a surge of intense emotion as the baby's head began to emerge. The final moments of delivery were filled with a mix of exhaustion and exhilaration.

With one final, determined push, the baby was born. The room erupted in cheers and applause as the baby let out a strong, healthy cry. Ethan's eyes filled with tears of joy as he saw their newborn child for the first time.

Mia, exhausted but overjoyed, looked at the baby with tears streaming down her face. The moment was surreal and beautiful, a culmination of months of anticipation and preparation. Dr. Simmons carefully placed the baby on Mia's chest, and the connection between mother and child was immediate and profound.

Ethan stood beside Mia, his hand resting gently on the baby's tiny back. "Welcome to the world, little one," he whispered, his voice choked with emotion.

The baby's cries soon softened as they were gently swaddled and examined by the nurses. Mia and Ethan took in the sight of their newborn, marveling at the tiny fingers, delicate features, and the overwhelming sense of love that filled the room.

As the initial excitement settled, the medical team continued their post-delivery checks and assisted with the transition to the recovery room. Mia and Ethan were guided through the process of bonding with their baby, and they took the time to marvel at the new addition to their family.

The first moments with their baby were a mix of wonder and tenderness. Mia and Ethan took turns holding and gazing at their newborn, their hearts overflowing with love and gratitude. The exhaustion of labor was quickly forgotten in the presence of their precious child.

As the day turned to night, Mia and Ethan found themselves in a state of contented disbelief. They had navigated the challenges of labor and delivery and were now holding their baby in their arms. The experience had been transformative, and they were filled with a sense of accomplishment and joy.

The arrival of their baby marked the beginning of a new chapter in their lives. Mia and Ethan looked forward to the journey ahead, eager to embrace the challenges and joys of parenthood. The labor and delivery experience had been a testament to their strength, love, and commitment to each other and their growing family.

With their baby peacefully resting in the nursery, Mia and Ethan took a moment to reflect on the incredible journey that had brought them to this point. They were ready to embrace the future with open hearts and eager anticipation, knowing that the love they shared would guide them through the adventures and challenges of parenthood.

As the first rays of dawn peeked through the hospital window, Mia and Ethan settled into their new reality as parents. The journey of labor and delivery had been a remarkable experience, and they were grateful for the support, care, and love that had surrounded them every step of the way.

Their lives had changed forever, and they were ready to embrace the joys and challenges of parenthood with open hearts and unwavering commitment. The arrival of their baby was the beginning of a beautiful new chapter, and Mia and Ethan were excited to embark on this journey together as a family.

Chapter 15: The First Days

The first days with their newborn were a whirlwind of emotions and adjustments for Mia and Ethan. The hospital had provided a cocoon of support and care, but now they were heading home, ready to embark on the next phase of their journey as a family.

The car ride from the hospital to their home was filled with a mix of excitement and nervousness. Mia sat in the back seat, holding their baby, while Ethan drove. The baby slept peacefully in the car seat, a small bundle of contentment amidst the excitement of their new reality.

As they pulled into their driveway, Ethan glanced in the rearview mirror, catching Mia's eye. "We're finally home," he said with a smile, his voice tinged with awe.

Mia nodded, her gaze fixed on the tiny face of their baby. "I can't believe it. This is really happening."

The transition from hospital to home was both exhilarating and overwhelming. Their home had been prepared meticulously for the baby's arrival, with the nursery ready and the house stocked with supplies. Yet, the reality of caring for a newborn set in quickly.

As they carried their baby inside, they were greeted by a quiet house. The nursery was pristine, with the crib set up and a cozy corner for feeding and changing. Mia and Ethan took their time settling in, setting up the baby's things, and organizing their own space.

The first night at home was a mixture of excitement and challenge. The baby's needs were constant, from feeding to changing to soothing. Mia and Ethan took turns attending to their baby's needs, learning to navigate the demands of parenthood in real time.

Mia found herself marveling at the small details of their baby's face, the delicate fingers, and the tiny sounds of contentment. Despite the exhaustion, she was captivated by the joy of having their baby with them.

Ethan, too, was struck by the profound sense of responsibility and love he felt. He took on tasks with a newfound sense of purpose, from preparing bottles to comforting the baby during the night.

As the days passed, Mia and Ethan began to establish a routine. They learned to read their baby's cues, understanding the signs of hunger, sleepiness, and discomfort. The early days were a learning experience, filled with moments of trial and error as they adjusted to the new rhythm of their lives.

One morning, as they sat in the living room with their baby nestled between them, Mia and Ethan shared a quiet moment of reflection.

"I never imagined it would be like this," Mia said softly, looking at their baby. "It's overwhelming, but it's also so wonderful."

Ethan nodded in agreement. "It's like everything else fades away when we're with our baby. It's just us and this little person."

The support of family and friends was a crucial element in their adjustment period. Joan and the rest of Mia's family were eager to help, offering meals, advice, and a listening ear. They visited often, bringing homemade dishes and checking in on Mia and Ethan's well-being.

Mia's parents were particularly involved, providing both practical assistance and emotional support. Joan often came over to help with household chores and to spend time with the baby, allowing Mia and Ethan to rest and recharge.

The advice and encouragement from their loved ones were invaluable, but Mia and Ethan also faced the challenge of establishing their own parenting style. They navigated differing opinions and advice with patience and grace, finding what worked best for their family.

The first few days were marked by moments of both triumph and frustration. The joys of witnessing their baby's first smiles and coos were tempered by the exhaustion of sleepless nights and the challenges of feeding and soothing.

Despite the challenges, Mia and Ethan found solace in their partnership. They supported each other through the ups and downs, sharing in the joys and responsibilities of parenthood. Their bond grew stronger as they navigated the early days together.

As they settled into their new routine, Mia and Ethan also found time to reflect on the support they had received from their community. The outpouring of love and encouragement from family and friends was a testament to the strength of their support network.

One afternoon, as Mia and Ethan took turns holding the baby, they shared their thoughts about the journey ahead.

"I feel like we're just beginning to scratch the surface," Mia said, her eyes shining with determination. "There's so much to learn and experience."

Ethan smiled, his hand resting gently on the baby's back. "We'll take it one day at a time. We've got each other, and that's the most important thing."

As the days turned into weeks, Mia and Ethan continued to adapt to the new dynamics of their lives. They embraced the challenges with resilience and optimism, finding joy in the small moments and milestones.

The first days with their baby were a time of profound change and growth. Mia and Ethan learned to balance their roles as parents with their own needs, finding ways to support each other and nurture their relationship.

They celebrated the small victories, from a successful feeding to a peaceful nap, and faced the challenges with determination and love. The early days were a testament to their strength as a couple and their commitment to their growing family.

As they settled into the rhythm of their new life, Mia and Ethan felt a deep sense of fulfillment. The arrival of their baby had transformed their lives in ways they had never imagined, and they were ready to embrace the journey ahead with open hearts and unwavering commitment.

The first days were just the beginning of a new chapter, and Mia and Ethan looked forward to the adventures and joys that awaited them as they continued to build their family together. With love, support, and a sense of wonder, they embraced the challenges and celebrated the triumphs of parenthood, ready to face the future as a family.

Chapter 16: Embracing the Future

With the initial whirlwind of welcoming their baby into the world behind them, Mia and Ethan began to settle into their new routine. The days blended into a rhythm of feedings, diaper changes, and tender moments of bonding. As they navigated the challenges of parenthood, they found themselves looking forward with a mix of excitement and anticipation for the future.

The house had transformed into a haven of warmth and comfort, a reflection of the new chapter in their lives. The nursery was filled with soft colors and gentle light, creating a peaceful space for their baby. Each corner of the house seemed to whisper the promise of new beginnings and cherished memories.

One evening, after a particularly peaceful day, Mia and Ethan found themselves sitting together on the couch, their baby sleeping contentedly in the crib nearby. They took a moment to relax and reflect on their journey.

"I can't believe how much has changed in such a short time," Mia said, her voice filled with wonder. "It feels like we've been on this incredible adventure."

Ethan nodded, his eyes filled with admiration. "It's been an amazing journey, and it's just beginning. There's so much to look forward to."

The couple took solace in the small victories and milestones they experienced with their baby. From the first smiles to the discovery of tiny fingers and toes, each moment was a reminder of the profound joy that parenthood brought.

They also faced the challenges with resilience. The sleepless nights and unpredictable schedules tested their patience and stamina, but they approached each obstacle with determination and teamwork. Their bond grew stronger as they navigated the ups and downs of parenting together.

Mia and Ethan were committed to creating a nurturing environment for their baby. They made an effort to establish routines that balanced their needs as individuals and as parents. They carved out time for themselves, whether it was a quiet evening together or a simple walk around the neighborhood, knowing that maintaining their connection was essential.

Their support network continued to play a vital role in their lives. Family and friends remained a constant source of encouragement and assistance.

Joan and Mia's parents frequently visited, offering practical help and sharing in the joys of watching their grandchild grow. Their support was a comforting reminder of the strong community surrounding them.

One sunny afternoon, Mia and Ethan decided to take their baby for a walk in the stroller. They strolled through the park, enjoying the fresh air and the tranquility of the outdoors. The experience was a welcome change of pace and an opportunity to bond as a family.

As they walked, Ethan glanced at Mia, his expression thoughtful. "I've been thinking about the future, about what we want for our family."

Mia smiled, appreciating the depth of the conversation. "Me too. I want to make sure we create a loving and supportive environment for our baby. I want them to feel cherished and secure."

Ethan nodded, his gaze focused on the path ahead. "I agree. I want us to stay connected, to keep growing as individuals and as a couple. I think that's important for our family."

The walk was a chance for Mia and Ethan to discuss their hopes and dreams for their baby's future. They talked about the values they wanted to instill, the experiences they hoped to share, and the way they envisioned their family evolving.

As the days turned into weeks, Mia and Ethan continued to adapt to their new roles. They made an effort to balance their responsibilities, finding joy in the small moments and celebrating the milestones along the way. The first smiles, the first coos, and the early interactions with their baby were treasured memories that they would cherish forever.

They also embraced the opportunities to grow as individuals. Mia pursued hobbies and interests that brought her joy, while Ethan took time to focus on his own passions. They supported each other's personal growth, understanding that maintaining their own well-being was essential for their family's happiness.

The couple made a point of setting goals and planning for the future. They discussed their aspirations, from career goals to personal development, and how they could achieve a balance between their ambitions and their responsibilities as parents.

One evening, as they sat together with their baby nestled between them, Mia and Ethan reflected on their journey. They looked at each other with a sense of accomplishment and hope for the future.

"I'm so grateful for everything we've experienced," Mia said softly. "It's been challenging, but it's also been incredibly rewarding."

Ethan smiled, his hand resting gently on their baby's back. "I feel the same way. We've come so far, and I'm excited for all the moments ahead."

As they embraced the future, Mia and Ethan remained focused on the values and principles that mattered most to them. They were committed to creating a loving, supportive, and nurturing environment for their baby. Their journey had just begun, and they were ready to face the adventures and challenges of parenthood with optimism and love.

The days ahead were filled with endless possibilities. Mia and Ethan looked forward to the experiences and milestones that awaited them, eager to build a future that was rich with love, connection, and joy. The road ahead was uncertain, but they were confident that, together, they could navigate the path with grace and strength.

In the quiet moments of their daily life, Mia and Ethan found contentment in the simple joys of parenthood. They celebrated the growth and development of their baby, cherished their time together as a family, and embraced the opportunities to create lasting memories.

As they continued to build their life together, Mia and Ethan remained grateful for the love and support that had guided them. Their journey as parents was just beginning, and they were excited to embrace the future with open hearts and unwavering commitment.

The arrival of their baby had transformed their lives in ways they had never imagined. With love, hope, and a deep sense of connection, Mia and Ethan looked forward to the adventures and joys that awaited them, ready to embrace the future and create a beautiful life for their growing family.

Epilogue

The morning sun poured through the window, bathing the nursery in a warm, golden light. Mia stood by the crib, gently rocking it with one hand while her other hand rested on her baby's tiny back. The room was filled with the soft sounds of morning—birds chirping outside, the distant hum of the city waking up, and the peaceful, rhythmic breathing of her sleeping child.

As she looked down at the baby nestled in the crib, a sense of profound contentment washed over her. It felt like just yesterday that she and Ethan had been anxiously preparing for the arrival of their little one, their hearts brimming with a mix of excitement and uncertainty. Now, as she watched their baby sleep peacefully, it was hard to believe how quickly the time had passed.

The journey from those early, sleepless nights to this tranquil morning had been filled with countless moments of joy, growth, and discovery. Each day had brought new challenges and triumphs, from the first coos and giggles to the late-night feedings and the first steps taken with wobbly determination. Mia and Ethan had navigated the highs and lows of parenthood with a deep sense of love and dedication, and their bond had grown stronger with each passing day.

The living room was adorned with family photos, capturing the milestones and memories of their journey. There was a picture of Ethan holding their baby for the first time, his face radiant with pride. Another showed Mia cradling their child in the hospital, a look of awe and wonder in her eyes. Each photograph told a story of love, support, and the beautiful transformation that had taken place in their lives.

Mia's thoughts drifted to the day she and Ethan had first learned of their pregnancy. The news had been unexpected, but it had brought with it a joy that had blossomed into a profound and enduring love. Their journey had been one of growth and discovery, as they learned to embrace the challenges and cherish the moments of triumph.

Ethan entered the room, his presence a comforting anchor in the midst of their new reality. He wrapped his arms around Mia, pulling her close. Together, they looked down at their baby, their hearts swelling with pride and gratitude.

"It's incredible how much our lives have changed," Ethan said softly, his voice filled with emotion. "I never imagined it would be like this, but I wouldn't trade it for anything."

Mia smiled, her eyes shining with love. "It's been an amazing journey, and it's only the beginning. I'm so grateful for every moment we've shared."

As they stood together, holding their baby between them, they reflected on the path they had traveled. They had faced challenges and embraced joys, and their love had grown in ways they had never anticipated. The unexpected blessing of their child had brought them closer together, and their family had become a source of strength and happiness.

The future stretched out before them, filled with endless possibilities. They were excited to watch their baby grow, to guide them through life's adventures, and to continue building a home filled with love and laughter. The journey ahead would undoubtedly bring new challenges, but Mia and Ethan were ready to face them with the same unwavering commitment and love that had guided them so far.

In the quiet of the nursery, as they watched their baby sleep, Mia and Ethan felt a deep sense of fulfillment. Their hearts were full of love and hope, and they were ready to embrace whatever the future had in store. The story of their unexpected joy had blossomed into a beautiful reality, and they looked forward to the countless moments of joy, discovery, and love that lay ahead.

As the sun continued to rise, casting its gentle light over the room, Mia and Ethan stood together, united in their love for their child and their commitment to their family. The journey had been extraordinary, and the future was filled with the promise of more beautiful moments to come. With hearts full of gratitude and anticipation, they embraced the new chapter of their lives, ready to face the adventures and joys that awaited them as a family.

By

Gabreille Vicky

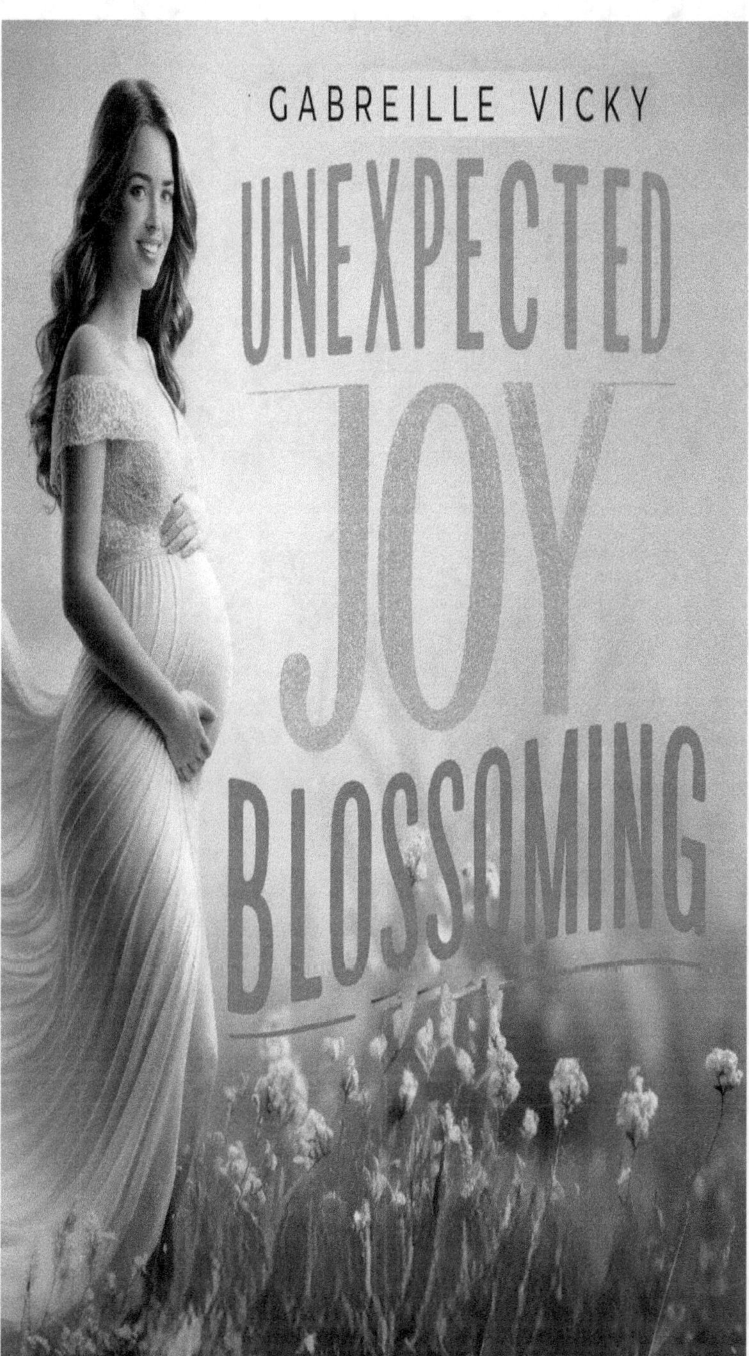

GABREILLE VICKY
UNEXPECTED
JOY
BLOSSOMING

www.ingramcontent.com/pod-product-compliance
Lightning Source LLC
Chambersburg PA
CBHW070837250726

48662CB00003B/1270